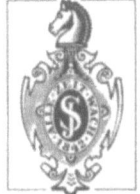

Hans Lassmann

Comparative Neuropathology of Chronic Experimental Allergic Encephalomyelitis and Multiple Sclerosis

With 37 Figures

Springer-Verlag Berlin Heidelberg GmbH 1983

Dr. med. HANS LASSMANN
Neurologisches Institut der Universität Wien,
Schwarzspanierstraße 17, A-1090 Wien IX

ISBN 978-3-642-45560-5   ISBN 978-3-642-45558-2 (eBook)
DOI 10.1007/978-3-642-45558-2

Library of Congress Cataloging in Publication Data
Lassmann, H. (Hans), 1949– Comparative neuropathology of chronic experimental allergic encephalomyelitis and multiple sclerosis. (Neurology series; 25) Bibliography: p. 1. Allergic encephalomyelitis – Addresses, essays, lectures. 2. Multiple sclerosis – Addresses essays, lectures. 3. Allergic encephalomyelitis – Animal models – Addresses, essays, lectures. 4. Pathology, Comparative – Addresses, essays, lectures. I. Title. II. Series. [DNLM: 1. Encephalomyelitis, Allergic – Pathology. 2. Multiple sclerosis – Pathology. W1 SC344 Bd. 25 / WL 360 L347c] RC370.L37 1983 616.8'32 83-4753

© by Springer-Verlag Berlin Heidelberg 1983
Softcover reprint of the hardcover 1st edition 1983

Typesetting: Druckservice K. Teichmann, 6901 Mauer

Foreword

For several decades the unsolved etiogenetic and therapeutic problems of multiple sclerosis have offered the strongest challenge to research in neurology. The hope of decisive theoretical and practical progress increased when an experimental model presenting far-reaching conformity of structural and pathogenetic features was developed, namely chronic relapsing experimental allergic encephalomyelitis (CREAE). During the past years, Dr. Lassmann has contributed substantially to the adaptation of this model with the aim of comprehensive evaluation, thoroughly following up his own ideas in numerous studies of individual aspects. The new possibility of continuous and detailed investigation of the clinical, morphological and immunological characteristics of temporal phase sequence of autoimmune demyelination has led to many new findings, corrections of former hypotheses, and, from correlated studies of human multiple sclerosis, a series of important data concerning, for example, early manifestations of demyelination, the range of so-called acute multiple sclerosis and the incidence of remyelination. Moreover, Dr. Lassmann has analysed several special problems which became definable in the course of his own studies or in collaboration with other groups, including the initial distribution of demyelinated foci, the cerebrospinal fluid phenomena and immunological findings in the nervous tissue. The results of these separate studies also led to a deeper understanding of demyelinating processes.

This monograph integrates these studies and summarizes their results. It is impressive how, through methodically extensive elaboration and through experimental analysis and follow-up of emergent problems the application of the one model of CREAE has both produced a representative survey of the current experimental realm and established a solid, in many respects conclusively demonstrated, and in relevant details new pathogenetic concept of the medical target of the research, the human disease multiple sclerosis.

Thus the book offers not only a complete report on the findings obtained from the CREAE model, but also an enlarged and improved interpretation of the complex process of multiple sclerosis. The information contained herein appears to constitute definite progress towards control of the fatal course of this disease.

Franz Seitelberger

Contents

1 Introduction

The pathogenesis of inflammatory demyelinating diseases and especially of multiple sclerosis has puzzled scientists of many medical disciplines during the past decades. Several different theories have been proposed regarding the pathogenetic factors responsible for, or involved in, the formation of the lesions. The most important still discussed in recent publications and reviews are autoimmunity (Lumsden 1971; Seitelberger 1967; Frick 1979; Lisak 1980), infection (Steiner 1931; Pette 1928; Waksmann 1980), vascular changes (Putnam 1935; Field 1979), and metabolic or toxic factors (Marburg 1906; Field 1979; Wolfgram 1979).

In spite of the large amount of research undertaken recently in immunology, virology, and biochemistry, pathogenetic theories of inflammatory demyelinating diseases are still largely based on the interpretation of the pathology of the lesions. This, however, raises the question of the pathology of these diseases – a question which at first seems inappropriate because of the large number of original case descriptions and reviews on this topic (Charcot 1868; Marburg 1906; Siemerling and Raeke 1914; Dawson 1916; Pette 1928; Hallervorden 1940; Seitelberger 1960, 1973; Jellinger 1969; Lumsden 1970; Oppenheimer 1976; Adams 1977).

It is now generally accepted that the main pathohistological characteristics of inflammatory demyelinating diseases are perivenous inflammation, selective (segmental) demyelination, and reactive gliosis. However, reviewing the literature and studying a large collection of multiple sclerosis (MS) cases, one is always astonished by the variable spectrum of the structural expression of the lesions in this disease. It includes extent of demyelination, topographical distribution of the lesions, extent of oligodendroglia destruction, remyelination, sclerosis and vascular pathology, and involvement of the peripheral nervous system.

The interpretation of this variability has been difficult up to now, because of the lack of an experimental model which not only fulfills the basic pathohistological criteria of MS but which in addition shows a similar large spectrum of structural changes in the lesions.

Experimental allergic encephalomyelitis (EAE) has been considered as an experimental model for human inflammatory demyelinating diseases since the earliest descriptions by Rivers et al. (1933) and Rivers and Schwentker (1935). This view was further supported by the introduction of reproducible models of chronic (Stone and Lerner 1965) and chronic relapsing EAE (Wisniewski and Keith 1977).

EAE, however, is a disease induced by active sensitization of susceptible animals with central nervous tissue in complete Freund's adjuvant, which is hardly comparable to disease induction in human MS. Furthermore, the disease duration, even in the most chronic models presently available, does not exceed 12–15 months after sensitization (Lassmann and Wisniewski 1979a) and seems to be related to the persistence of the sensitizing material at the inoculation site (Wisniewski et al. 1982).

In spite of these differences in etiology, the pathology of EAE closely mimics the tissue alterations described in human inflammatory demyelinating diseases (Alvord 1970; Raine et al 1974; Lassmann and Wisniewski 1979a). There is, however, still no detailed comparative pathohistological study of chronic EAE and MS available. Furthermore, the investigation of the sequence of events leading to the formation or influencing the structural expression of lesions in acute and chronic EAE may help us to understand the pathogenetic factors involved in the formation of inflammatory demyelinating lesions not only in experimental animals but also in humans.

2 The Spectrum of Inflammatory Demyelinating Diseases

For most clinicians, neuroimmunologists, and neurochemists studying the pathogenesis of multiple sclerosis, this disease is a clearly defined syndrome, characterized by a chronic relapsing or chronic progressive clinical course and by the presence of multifocal lesions in the central nervous system and well-defined immunological patterns in the cerebrospinal fluid and serum of patients. From the view point of neuropathologists, however, MS is only one member of a large family of closely related diseases, i.e., the inflammatory demyelinating diseases (Adams and Kubik 1952; v. Leyden 1880; Oppenheim 1914; Finkelnburg 1901; Marburg 1906; G. Peters 1958; Hallervorden 1940; Krücke 1973). These diseases include acute hemorrhagic leukoencephalomyelitis (Hurst 1941; Adams et al. 1948); acute perivenous (postinfectious, disseminated) leukoencephalomyelitis (Turnbull and McIntosh 1926–27); acute multiple sclerosis (Marburg 1906); and the chronic forms of MS (Charcot 1868), including neuromyelitis optica (Devic 1894; G. Peters 1970), concentric sclerosis (Balo 1928), and some forms of diffuse sclerosis (Schilder 1912). A similar spectrum of diseases can be induced experimentally by sensitization of susceptible animals with CNS tissue.

2.1 Experimental Models

Many different models of experimental allergic encephalomyelitis have been described during the past years; these depend on the sensitization procedures and the animals used in the experiments.

Acute ordinary EAE is the most frequent model induced by sensitization of susceptible animals with nervous tissue or myelin basic protein together with complete Freund's adjuvant (Morgan 1946; Alvord 1970). It is an acute monophasic disease, pathohistologically characterized by perivenous inflammation of mononuclear cells and a variable degree of perivenous demyelination, thus closely resembling the changes in acute perivenous leukoencephalitis.

Hyperacute EAE is induced by sensitization of very susceptible animal strains with central nervous system antigens using pertussis vaccine as adjuvant (Levine and Wenk 1965). The disease is also monophasic, and the onset of the disease is earlier than in acute ordinary EAE. The pathohistological changes, with massive alterations in the walls of small veins and venoles with extensive blood-brain barrier damage (Paterson 1976), migration of polymorphonuclear leukocytes into the perivascular tissue, and perivascular necrosis together with small hemorrhages, closely resemble the alterations described in acute hemorrhagic leukoencephalomyelitis in man (Levine 1971): Although the induction of the full picture of hyperacute EAE requires a special sensitization procedure, some overlap of the pathohistological features of hyperacute and ordinary EAE may be noted (Waksman and Adams 1962; Field and Raine 1969).

Other models in which acute EAE is modified by interference with the immune response or the target organ during the incubation period are acute necrotizing myelopathy (Levine and Sowinski 1976), an exceptionally severe form of EAE which is restricted to the spinal cord, and several models of localized EAE (Levine 1974).

Chronic progressive and chronic relapsing EAE differ from acute EAE by the large extent of demyelination. Most of the chronic demyelinating models of EAE have in common that:
1. Native CNS tissue is used for sensitization
2. High doses of antigen are used (up to 100 times the dose needed for the induction of acute EAE)
3. A very high amount of heat-inactivated mycobacterium is mixed to the adjuvant (5–10 mg/ml of encephalitogenic emulsion)

Several different models of chronic EAE have been described: Chronic EAE in monkeys was first described by Rivers et al. (1933). Pathological findings of large demyelinated lesions were noted; these were frequently localized in the periventricular white matter. Demyelination, although the main event, was accompanied by multiple foci of tissue necrosis. Furthermore, the inflammatory infiltrates were to a large extent composed of polymorphonuclear leukocytes (Rivers et al. 1933; Ferraro and Cazzullo 1948; Ravkina et al. 1978).

In Lewis rats McFarlin et al. (1974) reported a recurrent form of EAE, and the relapse of the disease followed 10–15 days after of the onset the acute episode. No further relapses of the disease were noted. Pathology revealed the presence of perivenous inflammation and demyelination similar in extent to that found in acute and subacute models of EAE. More recently we have sensitized Sprague Dawley rats with an antigen mixture identical to that used for induction of chronic relapsing EAE in guinea pigs (Wisniewski and Keith 1977). Most of the animals developed a chronic, frequently relapsing disease pattern. However, pathohistological findings in the majority of the animals showed the active disease in the chronic stage to be due to inflammatory demyelinating lesions in the peripheral nervous system (Lassmann et al. 1980a). Furthermore, lesional morphology in rats with chronic CNS disease differed in many respects from that found in chronic EAE in guinea pigs (Lassmann et al. 1980a, b). Both experiments, however, showed that the induction of chronic EAE is not dependent upon sensitization of juvenile animals with immature immune systems (McFarlin et al. 1974; Lassmann et al. 1980a).

4

In mice the induction of EAE is difficult and generally requires the additional use of *Bordetella pertussis* (Levine and Sowinski 1973, 1974; Bernard and Carnegie 1975). Nevertheless a chronic form of EAE has been observed in mice (Raine et al. 1980; Brown et al. 1981); the pathological changes in this model are, however, not yet fully described, and thus a comparison with other chronic EAE models and multiple sclerosis is difficult.

The models of chronic EAE in guinea pigs are at present most completely investigated pathohistologically (Freund et al. 1950; Stone and Lerner 1965); Raine et al. 1974; Snyder et al. 1975a; Wisniewski and Keith 1977, Lassmann and Wisniewski 1979b). Clinically a chronic progressive or chronic relapsing disease course is noted in the majority of the animals (Stone and Lerner 1965; Lassmann and Wisniewski 1979b). The pathological picture is dominated by the triad of inflammation, demyelination, and reactive gliosis. Immunologically these animals reveal in the chronic stage of the disease increased immunoglobulin levels in the CNS (Mehta et al. 1980, 1981) together with an increased IgG/albumen ratio and the presence of oligoclonal bands of immunoglobulins in brain extracts (Mehta et al. 1981) and in the cerebrospinal fluid (Karcher et al. 1982).

The clinical and pathohistological expression of the disease depends mainly upon the strain of animals, age at the time of sensitization, dose of CNS antigen, and route of inoculation used in the experiments (Stone et al. 1969; Lassmann and Wisniewski 1979a, b). Thus, when animals are sensitized according to the method of Wisniewski and Keith (1977), the majority of strain 13 guinea pigs follow a moderate or mild clinical course with many relapses also in the late chronic phase of the disease (100–500 days after sensitization). On the other hand, Hartley guinea pigs, sensitized in an identical way to the strain 13 animals, show a much higher mortality in the acute phase of the disease, a severe clinical course during the early chronic phase (40–100 days after sensitization, and only mild exacerbations during later stages.

In the model of chronic relapsing EAE, especially in Hartley and less pronounced in strain 13 guinea pigs (Wisniewski and Keith 1977), pathohistological changes closely resembling hyperacute, ordinary, and chronic demyelinating EAE can be seen. The pathological picture is dependent upon the time interval between sensitization and sampling of the animals and upon the severity of the disease at different time intervals after sensitization (Lassmann and Wisniewski 1978, 1979b; Lassmann et al. 1980b) In this model four stages of the disease may be distinguished. The *acute stage* (10–20 days after sensitization) is dominated by perivenous inflammation without demyelination. In most severely affected animals in this phase of the disease a pattern clossely resembling hyperacute EAE with perivenous tissue necrosis and massive accumulation of polymorphonuclear leukocytes can be found. The *subacute stage* (20–40 days after sensitization) may reveal two types of pathology: In animals with remission of the disease only few perivenous inflammatory infiltrates are noted without invasion of inflammatory cells into the CNS parenchyma and without demyelination. In animals with active disease in this phase the classical picture of perivenous leukoencephalitis is found with peri-venous inflammation and perivenous demyelination. The *early chronic stage* of the disease (40–100 days after sensitization) shows large demyelinated plaques in the white matter in animals with active disease. Oligodendrocytes are generally spared and rapid remyelination may occur. In the *late chronic stage* of the disease (100–200 days after sensitization) large demyelinated plaques are formed with intense fibril-lary gliosis, destruction and loss of oligodendrocytes, and slow or absent remyelina-tion.

2.2 Human Diseases

The clinical and pathohistological features of acute hemorrhagic leukoencephalo-myelitis, acute perivenous leukoencephalitis, and multiple sclerosis are well de-fined and will therefore not be discussed in detail in this chapter (for reviews see Hallervorden 1940; Adams and Kubik 1952). There is, however, some controversy about the definition of acute MS and the differences between this disease and acute perivenous leukoencephalitis or chronic MS. In the following chapters we will use the definition introduced by Marburg (1906), who characterized acute MS as follows: a rapidly progressing clinical disease course frequently combined with fever which leads to death of the patient within 3 weeks to 6 months after onset of the first clinical signs. One remission and relapse of the disease may sometimes be noted during the observation period. The pathology is dominated by the existence of large demyelinated plaques which contrast to the perivenous demyelination in acute perivenous leukoencephalomyelitis. Most of the plaques are active, with the presence of recent myelin degradation products at the plaque margins or in perivas-cular position. In addition, there are some peculiarities in acute MS lesions which distinguish them from typical chronic MS plaques. These differences include the extent of inflammation, demyelination oligodendroglia destruction, sclerosis, and peripheral nervous system involvement; these will be discussed in detail in the fol-lowing chapters.

The close relationship between different types of human inflammatory demye-linating diseases has already been described in detail (Adams and Kubik 1952). Especially transitional forms of acute hemorrhagic leukoencephalitis with acute disseminated (perivenous) leukoencephalitis (Krücke 1973) and between acute perivenous leukoencephalitis and acute and chronic MS have been documented (Adams and Kubik 1952; Marburg 1906; Siemerling and Raeke 1914; Fränkel and Jakob 1913; Pette 1928). These findings strongly indicate that multiple sclerosis is not a uniform disease but comprises several chronic variants of inflammatory de-myelinating diseases, a fact which should always be kept in mind in studying the immunological and etiopathogenetic factors responsible for the induction of this disease.

3 Allergic Encephalomyelitis in Humans

A disease closely resembling experimental allergic encephalomyelitis in animals has been found in humans as a complication following vaccination with brain tissue containing rabies vaccine (Jochwed 1925; Lesniowski 1931; Uchimura and Shiraki 1957). Most of the reported cases had a short clinical duration and histopathologically closely resembled the picture of acute EAE (Shiraki and Otani 1959; Shiraki 1968). More chronic cases with a disease duration of 1–5 months revealed large demyelinated plaques, especially in the periventricular white matter, the optic system, and the spinal cord (Uchimura and Shiraki 1957). The pathology of these chronic cases resembled in many respects that found in multiple sclerosis. There were, however, several differences between this disease and typical chronic MS. The lesions were relatively small compared with those in chronic MS, all lesions showed changes of active demyelination, and gliosis was comparatively mild. Furthermore, the perivenous inflammatory reaction and cellular density in demyelinating lesions were higher than generally found in active lesions of chronic MS. Minor differences were also found in lesional topography. The plaques in patients after rabies vaccination were mainly localized in the periventricular white matter and the optic system, whereas other CNS areas were only mildly affected and lesions in the gray matter were absent. Because of the structural aspects of demyelinating lesions this disease is thus more closely related to Marburg's type of acute MS (Marburg 1906) than to typical chronic MS.

These observations of acute and chronic inflammatory demyelinating diseases following rabies vaccination are interesting; however, they cannot be directly compared with experimental allergic encephalomyelitis, and a possible role of virus antigens in the pathogenesis of the disease cannot be definitely excluded.

Direct proof that experimental allergic encephalomyelitis may occur in humans has been described by Jellinger and Seitelberger (1958) and Seitelberger er al. (1958), in a case of inflammatory demyelinating disease which followed misguided treatment of a patient with lyophilized brain tissue. The pathology of this case was comparable to that described by Uchimura and Shiraki (1957) as chronic complication of rabies vaccination.

Although these studies clearly show that an inflammatory demyelinating disease with many similarities to multiple sclerosis may be induced in humans by autosensitization with CNS tissue, it has to be stressed that in none of the described cases did the disease last longer than 3–6 months after the last challenge with antigen. This indicates that a persistant antigenic stimulation is necessary to keep the disease active in the chronic stage. Similarly in chronic relapsing EAE the activity of lesions in the chronic stage of the disease correlates with the persistance of remnants of the sensitizing material at the inoculation site (Tabira et al. 1982; Wisniewski et al. 1982).

4 The Pathology of Inflammatory Demyelinating Lesions

There are several essential pathohistological criteria of inflammatory demyelinating lesions, which form the link between such diverse clinical syndromes as acute hemorrhagic leukoencephalomyelitis and multiple sclerosis. They include:
- The invariable presence of inflammation, predominantly affecting small veins and venoles of the central nervous system
- Selective and segmental demyelination, leaving other tissue elements of the central and peripheral nervous system unaffected and
- Reactive gliosis

In spite of basic consensus regarding these essential pathohistological criteria, many structural aspects of human and experimental inflammatory demyelinating lesions are variable and thus controversial. In the following chapters I will try to address these unresolved topics by comparing the pathology of the well-defined experimental model of EAE with the alterations found in human inflammatory demyelinating diseases.

4.1 Inflammatory Reaction

As it is expressed in the definition of inflammatory demyelinating diseases, inflammation in addition to demyelination is the most specific and important feature in pathology (Hallervorden 1940). The inflammatory infiltrates follow a perivenous pattern (Marburg 1906; Dawson 1916; Waksman 1960b), the inflammatory cells in general accumulate in the perivenous connective tissue spaces (Marburg 1906; Rivers et al. 1933; Hallervorden 1940; Ferraro and Cazzullo 1948), and in severe active lesions may also migrate into the perivascular CNS parenchyma (Hallervorden 1940; Jervis and Koprowski 1948). In general the infiltrates are composed of small and large mononuclear cells together with a variable amount of plasma cells (Marburg 1906; Halervorden 1940; Alvord 1970; Guseo and Jellinger 1975), although in certain members of human inflammatory demyelinating diseases like acute hemorrhagic leukoencephalitis (Hallervorden 1940) and in special models of EAE (Rivers et al. 1933; Ferraro and Cazzullo 1948; Waksman and Adams 1962; Levine and Wenk 1965), polymorphonuclear leukocytes may be numerous. In spite of this general consensus on the basic aspects of inflammation in inflammatory demyeelinating lesions, there are still many controversial opinions, especially regarding the time course, distribution, and cellular composition of inflammation in the lesions.

4.1.1 Inflammation in Experimental Allergic Encephalomyelitis

In acute EAE, initial inflammatory infiltrates in the CNS can be found as early as 5 days after sensitization (Waksman and Adams 1962). The time interval between challenge and inflammation in the CNS can be even shortened when damage of the blood-brain barrier is induced simultaneously with sensitization (Levine 1974), when sensitized lymphocytes are passively transferred (Paterson 1960; Aström and Waksman 1962), or when both experimental procedures are combined (Levine 1974). The extent of inflammation gradually increases with time after sensitization (Waksman and Adams 1962), reaching maximal intensity within the first days after onset of clinical disease. Inflammatory infiltrates in initial stages or mild subclinical forms of acute EAE are mainly confined to the meninges of the spinal cord and brain. There the infiltrates are not evenly distributed but restricted to small veins at the anastomosis of parenchymal and meningeal vessels. In more severely affected animals inflammation is generally also located in the CNS parenchyma in the form of perivenous inflammatory cuffs (Fig. 1a). Although the majority of inflammatory cuffs are located in the white matter, inflammatory changes in the gray mattter are also frequent. The predominance of meningeal inflammation together with insufficient sampling of tissue are the main reasons for the erroneous description of clinical disease in EAE in the absence of inflammatory infiltrates (Levine et al. 1975).

Similarly in chronic relapsing EAE (Wisniewski and Keith 1977) initial inflammatory infiltrates in variable intensity may be found as early as 7 days after sensitization regardless of the presence or absence of a later clinically expressed acute disease episode (Grundke-Iqbal et al. 1980; Lassmann, unpublished). During the acute stage of the disease, which can be noted in about 80 % of guinea pigs sensitized according to the procedure described by Wisniewski and Keith (1977), a similar pattern of inflammation as described above for acute EAE is observed (Lassmann and Wisniewski 1978, 1979b). When animals are followed beyond the stage of acute EAE several different patterns of inflammatory response can be found:

Animals with a single acute disease episode which is not followed by further relapses show perivenous inflammatory cuffs in the meninges and CNS parenchyma for at least 40–150 days after sensitization; the intensity of inflammatory reaction gradually decreases with time after sensitization. In animals with classical chronic relapsing or chronic progressive disease course the inflammatory response is highest during the acute/subacute stage of the disease (10–40 dps). In the early chronic phase (40–100 dps) inflammation is still pronounced although topographically more restricted than in the acute/subacute stage (Fig. 1c). In the late chronic phase

10

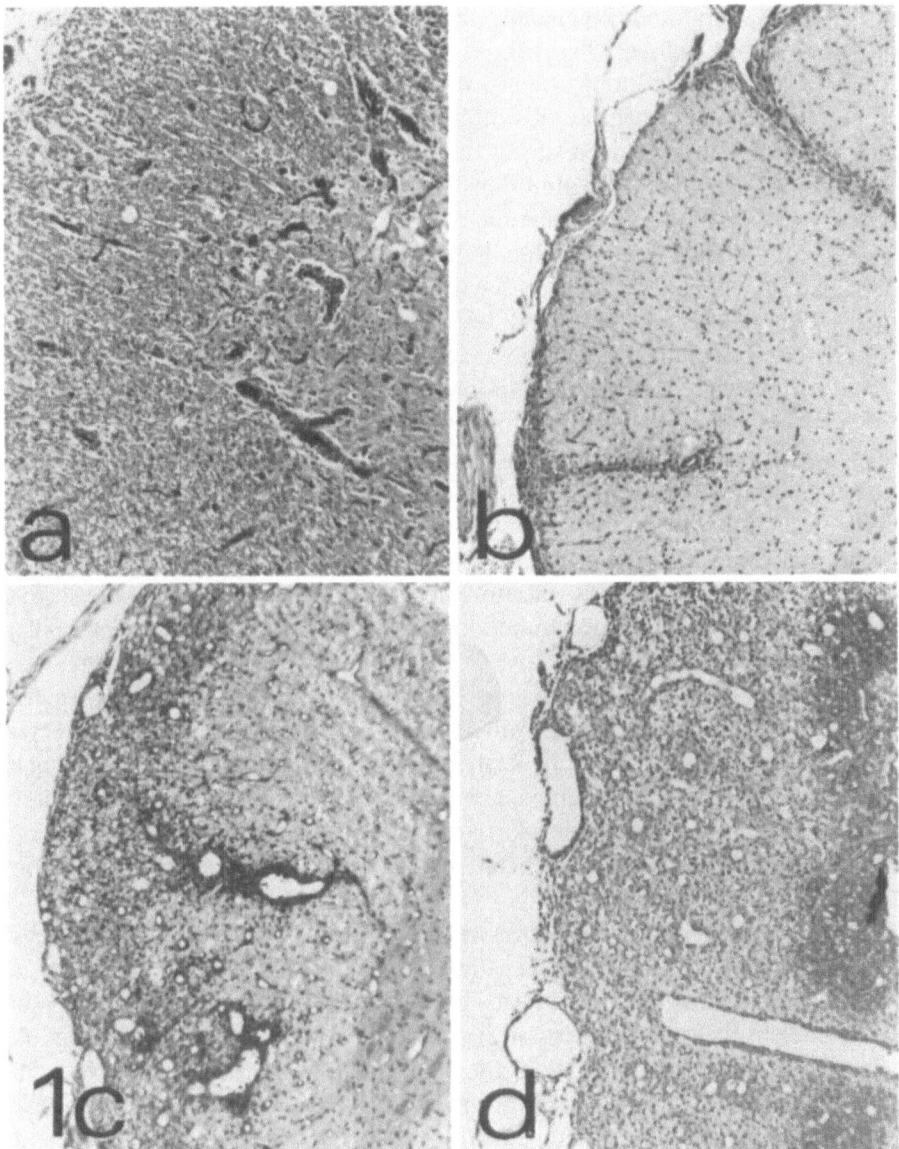

Fig. 1 a–d. Inflammatory reaction in different stages of chronic relapsing EAE. **a** Clinically active disease in the acute stage. Inflammatory reaction in the gray and white matter, localized around large and small veins. HE, x 60. **b** Severe clinical disease in the subacute stage. Inflammation is restricted to large drainage veins. HE, x 55. **c** Active disease in the early chronic stage. Large subpial zone of active demyelination. Inflammatory infiltrates are localized mainly around large drainage veins. HE, x 55. **d** Active disease in the late chronic stage. Large active demyelinating plaque. Inflammatory reaction is less pronounced than in Fig. 1c, in spite of massive active demyelination in the lesion. Lymphocytes and plasma cells mainly in the meninges and Virchow-Robin space of large drainage veins. HE, x 55

inflammatory infiltration is generally much less intense in spite of ongoing demyelination in these animals (Fig. 1d).

Animals sampled during a remission of the disease invariably show the presence of inflammatory perivenous infiltrates (Fig. 1b). During actively demyelinating episodes in chronic relapsing EAE, perivenous inflammatory cells are in general more numerous and more densely packed than with inactive lesions. Some inflammatory cells may penetrate the perivascular or subpial glia limitans and invade the underlying nervous tissue. In these lesions, however, small lymphocytes und plasma cells in the majority stay in their perivenous position. Only few of them, especially in most fulminant lesions, can be found within the CNS parenchyma. On the contary large mononuclear cells and debris containing phagocytes migrate more freely between the lesional tissue and the perivenous conncective tissue space. Thus the majority of inflammatory cells within the lesion itself are phagocytes. In recent lesions these debris-containing phagocytes are scattered throughout the whole demyelinating plaque (Fig. 1c, d), but at later time intervals after the onset of plaque formation they accumulate in perivenous connective tissue spaces, in the meninges, and also around small capillaries. As will be discussed below this pericapillary accumulation of macrophages during the stage of debris removal seems to be an important mechanism for the induction of capillary fibrosis in chronic EAE.

The number of large mononuclear cells in the inflammatory infiltrates in actively demyelinating lesions together with the passage of debris-containing phagocytes through the glia limitians is variable in individual inflammatory demyelinating lesions in EAE, especially when plaques in different animal species are compared with each other. As an example this macrophage response in active lesions is much more intense in guinea pigs than in rats, even when plaques of similar size are compared.

Another interesting aspect of distribution of inflammatory infiltrates in EAE can be obtained by comparing the pathology of acute with typical chronic EAE lesions. During the acute disease stage (10–20 dps) the distribution of inflammatory cells is relatively even, involving all segments of veins up to the smallest venoles (Fig. 1a). In typical chronic lesions the pattern of inflammation is more focal. Inflammatory infiltrates are mainly arranged in the connective tissue space of the large drainage veins in the meninges and in the chorold plexus, and the individual inflammatory cuffs have a higher cellularity than in acute EAE (Fig. 1b–d). Small venoles which are not surrounded by a Virchow-Robin space are generally free of inflammation. This changing pattern in the distribution of inflammatory infiltrates is one of the reasons for the topographical distribution of inflammatory demyelinating lesions in chronic EAE, as areas with high lesional incidence are simultaneously areas with a high density of large drainage veins (the periventricular white matter and the lateral column of the spinal cord, Lassmann et al. 1981a, b).

The inflammatory cuffs in acute as well as chronic EAE are predominantly composed of lymphocytes and large mononuclear cells. With chronicity of the disease beginning after the 20th–30th day after sensitization an increasing number of plasma cells is found in the lesions (Grundke-Iqbal et al. 1980). Polymorphonuclear leukocytes may be present, especially in early stages of severe acute lesions. Their number depends upon the species of animals used for the experiments and upon the type of sensitization (Levine 1974). They are most frequent in monkeys, less frequent in guinea pigs, and nearly absent in rats and rabbits following sensitization with CNS tissue in complete Freund's adjuvant (Rivers et al. 1933; Ferraro and Cazzullo 1948; Waksman and Adams 1962; Lassmann and Wisniewski 1978). A few polymorphonuclear leukocytes may also be seen during the first days after onset of a severe clinical relapse in the chronic stage of EAE in guinea pigs (Lassmann and Wisniewski 1978). It is, however, interesting to note that in the model for chronic relapsing EAE in guinea pigs, even in animals suffering from hyperacute EAE in the acute stage of the disease, granulocytes always follow the appearance of mononuclear infiltrates and are highest in numbers not earlier than 2–3 days after clinical onset of the disease (Grundke-Iqbal et al. 1980; Lassmann and Wisniewski 1979b). Thus in these hyperacute lesions the occurrence polymorphonuclear leukocytes seems to be a secondary event following the primary typical mononuclear infiltrates of EAE. The secondary nature of granulocyte infiltration in this model in animals with hyperacute EAE is further indicated by the perivascular deposition of high amounts of immunoglobulins and complement in the lesions (Grundke-Iqbal et al. 1980). A similar sequentialy study of the development of classical hyperacute EAE (Levine and Wenk 1965) is still missing. The composition of the mononuclear cell infiltrate is more difficult to evaluate. The presence of B-lymphocytes and plasma cells has been documented by immunofluorescence (Ridley 1963; Grundke-Iqbal et al. 1980; Ackermann et al 1981) and by electron microscopy (Snyder et al. 1975a; Lassmann et al. 1980b). The relative proportion of B cells and plasma cells increases with chronicity of the disease (Grundke-Iqbal et al. 1980; Lassmann et al. 1980b). "Early (active) T-cells" have been shown to decrease in the circulation with the onset of clinical disease in acute EAE and at the same time to appear in the meningeal infilrates (Traugott et al. 1978). Similar fluctuations in this cells population have been documented with the onset of a relapse in chronic EAE (Traugott et al. 1979). This contrasts to the behavior of B-cells, as up to now no fluctuations have been noted which correlate with disease activity in acute and chronic EAE. Immunofluorescence revealed the presence of T cells within the white matter of EAE animals at the onset of a relapse (Traugott et al. 1981; Traugott et al. 1982a). A considerable proportion of inflammatory infiltrates in active lesions are, however, large mononuclear cells of probable monocyte origin (Smith and Waksman 1969) and macrophages.

In EAE there can be hardly any doubt that inflammation always precedes demyelination. In large chronic lesions a pattern may sometimes be found in singular sections where no inflammation is present in spite of ongoing demyelination. In these lesions, however, classical perivenous cuffs are found when serial sections are studied.

4.1.2 The Inflammatory Response in Human Inflammatory Demyelinating Diseases

It is now well established that the inflammatory reaction in acute hemorrhagic leukoencephalitis and in acute perivenous leukoencephalomyelitis is very similar if not identical to that found in hyperacute or acute ordinary EAE (Alvord 1970, Levine 1971). There is still some controversy about similarities and dissimilarities between inflammation in chronic EAE and MS.

In multiple sclerosis perivenous inflammatory infiltrates composed of lymphocytes, plasma cells, large mononuclear cells, and macrophages are regularly observed (Anton and Wholwill 1912; Marburg 1936; Pette 1928; Lumsden 1970; Guseo and Jellinger 1975; Prineas and Wright 1978). In a study of 143 autopsy cases of MS (Guseo and Jellinger 1975) inflammatory infiltrates were found in 60% of total cases and in 74% of actively demyelinating cases. MS cases without perivenous inflammation were either inactive (burned out) or were pretreated with immunosuppressive therapy. However, there seemed to be a few examples where ongoing demyelination in presumably untreated cases was found in the absence of inflammatory infiltrates. There are several aspects which cast doubt upon this interpretation. Tissue sampling in this study was limited and thus insufficient to exclude definitely the presence of inflammation. Furthermore, exact information regarding pretreatment schedules is frequently no longer available in retrospective studies. In addition, actively demyelinating lesions were determined by the presence of sudanophilic myelin degradation products within the lesions. As will be discussed below this is not an accurate criterion for determining the extent of active demyelination. Thus there is so far no hard evidence for the occurrence of actively demyelinating lesions in the absence of inflammation, although it cannot be definitely excluded in chronic MS.

More difficult in chronic MS is to prove the primary nature of inflammation, i.e., that inflammation always precedes demyelination and is not a reactive alteration due to tissue damage. As standardized sampling of cases during plaque formation is not possible, the main support for the primary nature of inflammation in this disease comes from the study of acute MS cases. In these cases a continuous transition of the classical perivenous inflammatory lesions of acute disseminated leukoencephalitis into typical MS plaques is regularly found (Marburg 1906; Dawson 1916; Seitelberger 1973; Krücke 1973).

The intensity of the inflammatory reaction is very high in acute disseminated leukoencephalitis and in acute MS, whereas in cases of chronic MS inflammation is much less pronounced, even in active ones (Guseo and Jellinger 1975). However, the number of inflammatory cells in chronic inactive MS cases, if calculated per cubic milliliter of tissue, is still high: 200–400 cells/mm^3 in unaffected white matter and 1722 cells/mm^3 in plaque tissue (Prineas and Wright 1978). As many of these cells were plasma cells, they may be responsible for the elevated immunoglobulin levels found in chronic MS lesions (Prineas and Wright 1978). However,

14

these counts based on very few samples must be interpreted with caution as the number of inflammatory cells within chronic MS plaques varies from case to case and even from plaque to plaque within the same case (Guseo und Jellinger 1975).

The distribution of inflammatory cells in acute perivenous leukoencephalomyelitis and MS shows a similar pattern to that described above in acute and chronic EAE respectively. Whereas in acute perivenous leukoencephalomyelitis inflammatory infiltrates are more evenly arranged around all segments of the venous vascular tree, in chronic MS inflammation is focal, predominantly affecting large drainage veins (Seitelberger 1973). Lymphocytes and plasma cells in MS plaques are generally localized in a perivenous position. Only in severe actively demyelinating lesions does the inflammatory process pass the glia limitans and disperse into the neural parenchyma (Hallervorden 1940). Although some small lymphocytes and plasma cells have been documented light and electron microscopically within the demyelinating lesions themselves (Sluga 1969; Lumsden 1970; Guseo and Jellinger 1975; Prineas and Wright 1978), they are present only in small numbers compared with the perivenous infiltrates. The hypercellularity of active MS plaques is mainly due to phagocytes. Although it is well known that a variable but minor proportion of debris may be degraded in astrocytes (Marburg 1906; Seitelberger 1960), the precise origin of the so-called "gitter cells," which remove the majority of debris in MS lesions, is not yet defined. This is so not only for MS but also for most other human and experimental conditions like Wallerian degeneration, trauma, or inflammatory diseases where a variable involvement of hematogenous cells versus local "microglia" in the removal of debris has been shown (for review, see Oehmichen 1978). The presence of T cells in MS plaques has also been shown histochemically (Traugott and Raine 1982b).

According to the above-described observation in chronic relapsing EAE, a good indicator for the hematogenous origin of phagocytes is the perivascular (pericapillary) accumulation of debris-containing cells in the stage of debris removal, together with the observation of these cells penetrating the perivascular glia limitans. Such observations have been made, although infrequently, in plaques in chronic MS (Prineas and Wright 1978). In acute MS, which is characterized by a higher intensity of inflammatory reaction compared with chronic cases (Marburg 1906), the perivenous and pericapillary accumulation of debris-containing cells is also much more pronounced.

In conclusion several common essential patterns regarding the inflammatory reaction in human inflammatory demyelinating diseases and different forms of experimental allergic encephalomyelitis can be extrapolated:
- The primary nature of inflammation in the disease in the sense that inflammation always precedes demyelination is well established in EAE and acute disseminated leukoencephalitis and acute MS. In chronic MS there is no hard evidence available that demyelination may occur in the absence of inflammation. This negative evidence, however, cannot be regarded as definite proof for the essential nature of inflammation in this condition.

- The distribution of inflammatory infiltrates changes with chronicity of the disease. In acute lesions (acute disseminated leukoencephalitis and acute EAE) inflammation involves all segments of veins including the smallest venoles, whereas in chronic EAE and MS infiltrates are arranged mainly around large drainage veins. This changing pattern seems to be partly responsible for the differences in lesional distribution in acute perivenous leukoencephalitis compared with MS (Seitelberger 1973).
- The inflammatory process is mainly confined to the perivenous connective tissue in the parenchyma and the meninges. Phagocytes pass the perivascular and superficial glia limitans easily in active lesions. However, only a very small proportion of lymphocytes and plasma cells can be found within the demyelinating lesion itself. It is not clear at present whether these cells represent the small fraction of specifically sensitized immunocompetent cells (Kosunen et al. 1963; Smith and Waksman 1969) or whether lymphocytes and plasma cells involved in the demyelinating process act from a distance via soluble mediators (as suggested by Arnason et al. 1969; Bornstein and Iwanami 1971; Lumsden 1971; Wisniewski and Bloom 1975) and not through a direct cellular attack on myelin.

4.2 Vascular Pathology

Changes in the structural organization of the vascular wall are a frequent finding, following a wide variety of CNS injuries like trauma, hypertension, neoplasms, inflammation, etc. (Spielmeyer 1922; Stochdorph and Meesen 1957). It is thus not surprising to find pronounced changes in the vascular architecture in chronic relapsing EAE and MS in diseases with persistent CNS inflammation for several months to years.

4.2.1 Vascular Pathology in EAE

Vascular alterations in EAE can be divided into acute forms, present in active lesions, and chronic forms, in inactive repaired plaques. In active lesions vascular changes consist mainly of cellular infiltration of veins and venoles (Waksman 1960) and perivascular accumulation of inflammatory cells and serum components (Paterson 1976; Ridley 1963; Pette et al. 1965; Oldstone and Dixon 1968; Simon and Anzil 1974) (Fig. 2a, b). In addition, in animals with severe inflammatory infiltration of the parenchyma during the stage of debris removal, macrophages may accumulate not only around veins and venoles but also around capillaries (Fig. 2a). Furthermore, in most severe lesions, thrombosis or rupture of small venoles can be sometimes found together with the appearance of perivenous hemorrhages (Ferraro and Cazzullo 1948) (Fig. 2e, f). In chronic inactive lesions the main alteration in the vascular walls is the increase of connective tissue especially around small venoles (Snyder et al. 1975b). In addition, a variable extent of capillary fibrosis may be found, which is most pronounced in areas of the CNS where active lesions are accompanied by intense pericapillary accumulation of debris-containing phagocytes (especially in spinal cord lesions in guinea pigs) (Figs. 2c, 3). In other lesions, e. g., in the rat brain where inflammatory infiltrates during the active stage are less pronounced and myelin degradation is performed to a large extent in local cells, capillary fibrosis is slight or absent (Fig. 2d).

Capillary fibrosis is combined with profound changes of the vascular architecture. The endothelium is separated from the perivascular glia limitans by a connective tissue space containing large amounts of collagen together with some fibroblasts and mononuclear cells (Fig. 3). An increased number of endothelial transport vesicles (Snyder et al. 1975b) may be the structural correlate of blood-brain barrier damage found in these vessels (Kristensson and Wisniewski 1977). In addition, endothelial fenestrae have been described in the vessels in chronic EAE lesions (Snyder et al. 1975b), although in other studies this finding has not been confirmed (Kristensson and Wisniewski 1977). This discrepancy may be explained by recent studies by Palade et al. (1979), which showed that endothelial fenestrae are not a static feature of endothelial cells but represent a structural expression of enhanced vesicular transendothelial transport. Fibrosed capillaries in chronic EAE lesions are similar to those found in the area postrema under normal conditions. Furthermore, this type of capillary pathology is not unique for EAE, but can also be found in many other pathological conditions of the brain, especially in those which are accompanied by chronic edema (Spielmeyer 1922; Stochdorph and Meesen 1957; Snyder et al. 1975b).

An increased vascular density can be found in chronic EAE lesions, but there are not quantitative data available proving the occurrence of vascular sprouting in EAE lesions. Thus, the increased vascular density may just be due to shrinkage of the parenchyma following plaque formation.

Vascular changes in EAE are clearly secondary events dependent in their severity upon the intensity of the inflammatory reaction during the active stage of the lesion. However, severe vascular changes by affecting the blood-brain barrier permeability may aggravate tissue damage and may facilitate the formation of new lesions.

Fig. 2 a–f. Vascular pathology in different models of chronic relapsing EAE **a** Active lesion in the guinea ▷ pig (Hartley) spinal cord. Massive accumulation of large mononuclear cells and macrophages around all vessels in the lesion, including capillaries. Toluidine blue, x 350. **b** Active lesion in the rat (Sprague Dawley) cerebellar white matter. Inflammatory cells are restricted to veins and venoles. Toluidine blue, x 350. **c** Inactive demyelinated plaque in the guinea pig spinal cord with extensive capillary fibrosis. Toluidine, x 350. **d** Inactive (remyelinated) lesion in the rat cerebellar white matter. Absence of capillary fibrosis. Toluidine blue, x 350. **e** Active lesion in the guinea pig centrum semiovale. Occlusion of small vessel. Toluidine blue, x 300. **f** Adjacent area of the same lesion. Scattered erythrocytes in the lesion. Intense protoplasmatic glia reaction. Toluidine blue, x 600

Fig. 3. Capillary fibrosis in demyelinated plaques in the guinea pig spinal cord. Inactive lesion with initial ▷▷ remyelination. EM, x 985

17

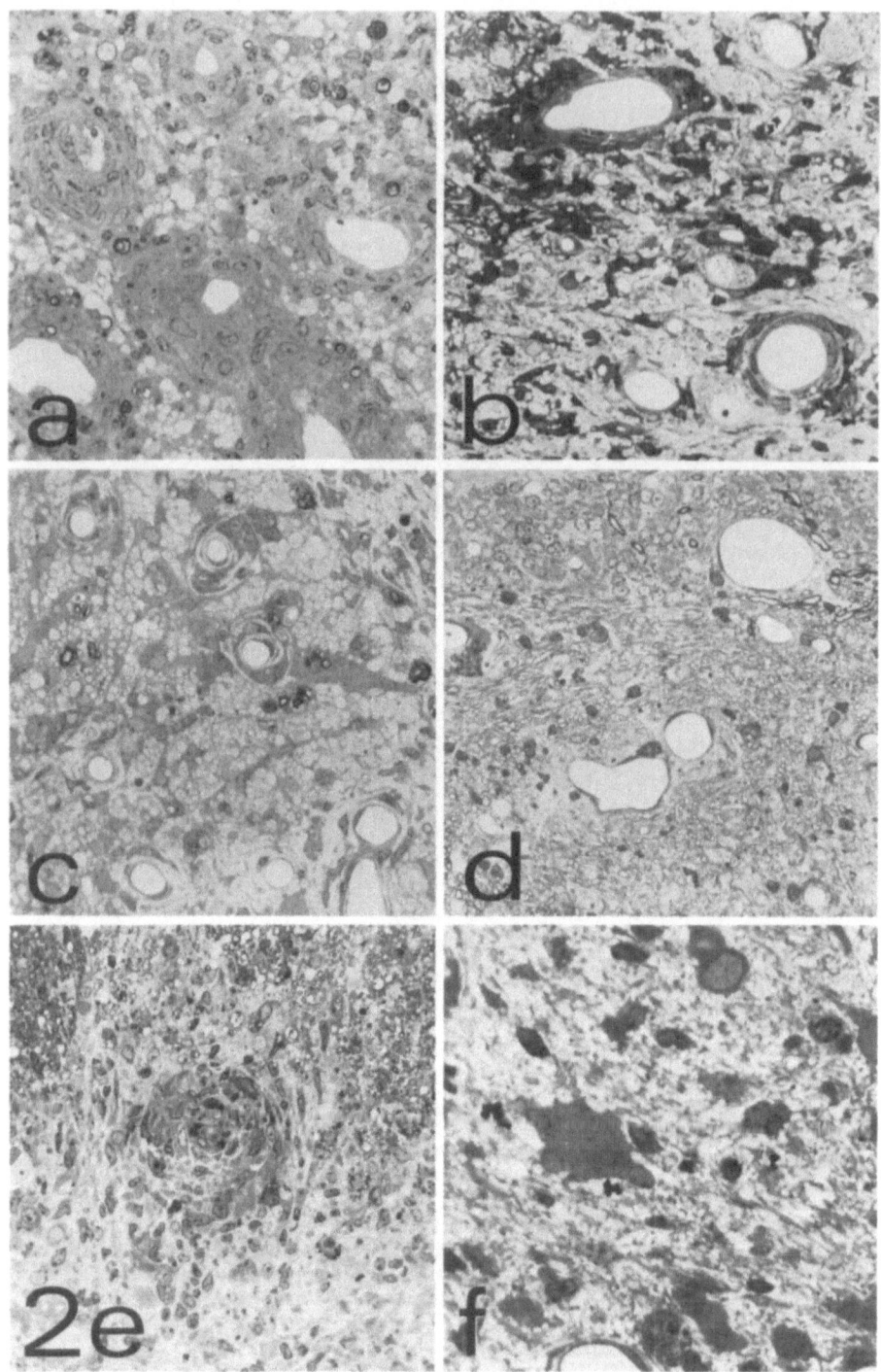

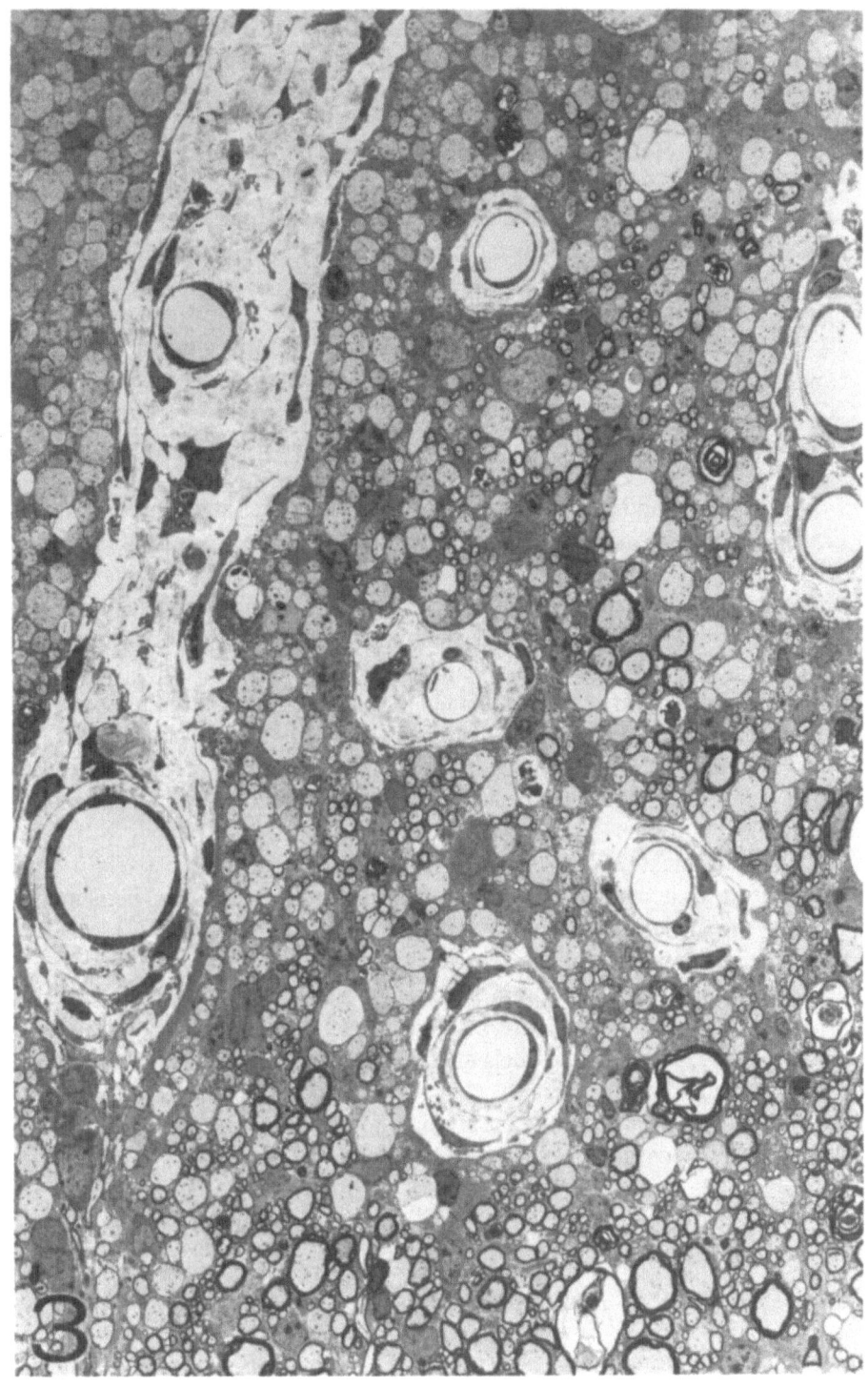

4.2.2 Vascular Pathology in Multiple Sclerosis

The occurrence of vascular alterations similar to those described above has been noted in nearly all light microscopic studies on MS pathology (Lumsden 1970). The observation of small venous thrombi and small perivenous hemorrhages in active MS plaques (Siemerling and Raeke 1914) has led to the concept that the main pathogenetic factor in this disease is the occlusion of small veins and that tissue damage is a result of coalescence of small perivenous ischemic lesions (Putnam 1935). Although the primary nature of venous thrombosis in MS pathogenesis has been ruled out by relatively low incidence of this alteration, by detailed studies of all stages of plaque formation and by the selective nature of myelin destruction (Marburg 1906, Dawson 1916; Lumsden 1970), it is still unresolved to what extent occlusion or damage to small drainage vessels may secondarily contribute to the lesional growth, especially in cases of concentric sclerosis (Field 1979; Courville 1970).

The incidence and intensity of chronic vascular changes like perivenous and pericapillary fibrosis is variable from case to case (Lumsden 1970). Suzuki et al. (1969) pointed out that vascular changes were absent in chronic subcortical plaques. On the other hand, Prineas and Wright (1978) noted intense perivascular fibrosis, however, they did not distinguish between small venoles and capillaries. In our experience pericapillary fibrosis may be pronounced in spinal cord and periventricular lesions whereas it is virtually absent in the subcortical white matter of the brain hemispheres and the cerebellum. Comparable with the findings in chronic relapsing EAE intense pericapillary fibrosis is found mainly in the same areas where pericapillary accumulation of phagocytes is pronounced in active lesions (Lassmann et al. 1981f).

Recently Prineas (1979) described the formation of lymphatic vessels in the enlarged perivascular connective tissue spaces in chronic MS plaques. Similar observations were made on a light microscopic level by Spielmeyer (1922), who described the formation of lymphatic channels and chamber systems in fibrosed CNS vessels not only in MS but also in all other diseases which were accompanied by pronounced perivascular increase of connective tissue. It is not yet clear, however, whether these lymphatic channels are connected with a lymphatic system comparable to that present outside the central nervous system. This question is especially interesting because of the observed lymph drainage from the CNS compartment into the cervical lymph nodes (Oehmichen 1978).

4.3 Blood-Brain Barrier

The blood-brain barrier (BBB) regulates the exchange of substances between the blood and the central nervous system (Ehrlich 1885; Goldman 1913; for reviews, see Lee 1971; Rapoport 1976). It thus plays a central role in the induction and propagation of inflammation as well as in the exchange of antigens, inflammatory mediators, and toxic metabolites between the CNS compartment and the circulation. The structure and physiological properties of the BBB, the blood-cerebrospinal fluid-barrier, and the cerebrospinal fluid-brain barrier have been extensively reviewed in the past years (Lee 1971; Rapoport 1976; Brightman et al. 1970; Brightman 1977), and therefore only a few aspects which are most relevant for the understanding of EAE pathogenesis will be discussed here.

4.3.1 Blood-Brain Barrier and Blood-CSF Barrier Leakage
Under Physiological Conditions

The blood-brain barrier is not an absolute but a partially permeable barrier, this allowing the passage of proteins and the establishment of an equilibrium of proteins between the serum and the CNS compartment under physiological conditions (Felgenhauer 1974; Tourtellotte et al. 1980). This "physiological leakage" occurs mainly via small caliber arterioles of the CNS parenchyma (Westergaard and Brightman 1973). Similarly a slow active transport of proteins from the CSF into the circulation has been found (Klatzo et al. 1964; Becker et al. 1968; Wagner et al. 1974; Van Deurs 1977), which is performed predominantly via small postcapillary venoles (Lassmann et al., unpublished). Thus, BBB damage is a quantitative phenomenon due to an increase in protein exchange between the CNS compartment and circulation which exceeds the physiological exchange rate. Meningeal vessels under normal conditions are more easily permeable for serum proteins than vessels in the CNS parenchyma (Waksman 1960a; Lee 1971). This may explain to some extent the frequent occurrence of inflammatory infiltrates in the meninges in EAE.

Another interesting aspect of BBB function is the effect of biogenic amines in BBB permeability, as these substances play an important role in affecting the permeability of blood vessels in the initial stages of inflammation in peripheral organs.

In the brain, however, biogenic amines seem to play only a minor role in affecting BBB permeability (Edvinson and McKenzie 1977). Both histamine and serotonin may induce only a minor increase in BBB permeability (Gross et al. 1981), probably by increasing the intravascular pressure and by reduction of blood flow in cerebral venoles (Westergaard 1975). A contraction of endothelial cells in venoles with opening of the interendothelial tight junction, leading to massive leakage of serum proteins, which can be induced by histamine in muscle tissue (Simionescu et al. 1978), has not been observed in the central nervous system.

4.3.2 The Diffusion of Proteins in the Extracellular Space of the Brain

Inflammation in the CNS in an autoimmune disease like EAE may be sustained by two different mechanisms: by the diffusion of soluble antigens to the vascular wall or by the migration of cells and the diffusion of soluble inflammatory mediators into the CNS parenchyma. Both mechanisms require the spread of proteins or other macromolecules in the extracellular space of the CNS along a considerable distance. Serum proteins which have passed the endothelial barrier in the brain in general may penetrate into the CNS tissue (Brightman 1965; Brightman et al. 1970; Van Deurs and Amtorp 1978). The size of the molecules is only a relative limiting factor in penetration, as even large molecules like ferritin (mol. wt: 650 000) may spread in the extracellular space of the brain (Brightman 1965).

Another factor which governs the mobility of molecules in the extracellular space of the brain is their molecular charge (Friedemann und Elkeles 1934; Waksmann 1960a). As an exemple kationized peroxidase with an isoelectric point close to that of myelin basic protein is able to diffuse from the cerebrospinal fluid into the spinal cord tissue only when applied in sufficiently high concentration (Kitz et al., in preparation). Furthermore, the diffusion is slower, and the kationic tracer is retained much longer in the CNS parenchyma than its neutral counterpart (Kitz et al., in preparation). Although it is still open whether myelin basic protein behaves similar to kationized peroxidase, these experiments indicate that the diffusion of charged molecules in the brain extracellular space is more restricted than that of neutral proteins.

4.3.3 Mechanisms and Structural Correlates of Blood-Brain Barrier Damage

Blood-brain barrier damage may occur by two different mechanisms: by the disturbance of the integrity of the endothelial lining via destruction of endothelial cells or opening of interendothelial tight junctions, and by increase of active transendothelial transport.

Disturbance of the integrity of the endothelium is rare and occurs mainly in early stages following CNS trauma and to some extent also in areas with severe inflammatory infiltrates of cerebral vessels. This type of damage generally leads to extensive perivascular accumulation of serum proteins.

Increase in active transendothelial transport is more commonly found as a mechanism of BBB damage. The structural correlate of this type of BBB damage is the increase in endothelial transport vesicles, the formation of transendothelial channels, and in rare instance the formation of endothelial fenestrae (Palade et al 1979; Vorbrodt et al. 1981). Increased active transport is found in a large variety of pathological conditions of the brain including intoxications, inflammatory diseases, and trauma, and is mainly characterized by leakage of albumin and immunoglobulins, but only minor or absent perivascular fibrin deposition.

4.3.4 The Blood-Brain Barrier in Experimental Allergic Encephalomyelitis

Increased permeability of cerebral vessels is a very early feature of EAE. It occurs before onset of clinical disease in acute EAE (Oldstone and Dixon 1968; Daniel et al. 1981). There ist still, however, some controversy as to whether it precedes the occurrence of inflammatory infiltrates. This aspect is difficult to resolve, as the absence of inflammatory infiltrates in leaking vessels can only be proven by serial section studies. In isolated pia mater preparations from animals before the onset of EAE, pronounced BBB leakage for IgG through meningeal vessels was restricted to vascular segments surrounded by inflammatory cuffs (Kitz et al. 1981). However, more detailed studies with different tracers and tracer concentrations are necessary to clarify whether in the incubation period of EAE in the absence of inflammation there is an increased transport rate for proteins through the endothelia of normal vessels which exceeds that found in unsensitized animals.

The extent of BBB damage in acute EAE is variable, depending upon the model studied (Oldstone and Dixon 1968; Pette et al. 1965; Paterson 1976). In ordinary acute EAE BBB damage, although invariably present, is relatively mild in comparison to hyperacute EAE. In the latter massive perivascular accumulation of all serum proteins including fibrin deposition is observed together with extensive perivascular accumulation of polymorphonuclear leukocytes and sometimes small perivenous hemorrhages (Grundke-Iqbal et al. 1980).

Tracer studies (Lampert and Carpenter 1965; Hirano et al. 1970) revealed that proteins mainly passed the barrier together with inflammatory cells through gaps in the endothelial lining. There is, however, also increased endothelial transport in vascular segments adjacent to sites of cellular passage (Hirano et al. 1970). Following recovery of animals from acute EAE some increased permeability of affected vessels may persist for a long time in spite of the absence of perivascular inflammatory infiltrates.

Similarly in chronic relapsing EAE massive leakage of serum proteins through cerebral vessels is found during the acute stage of the disease (10–20 dps; Grundke-Iqbal et al. 1980). In agreement with previous studies on models of acute EAE, the extent of BBB damage is dependent upon the histological appearance of the lesions with the most pronounced perivascular accumulation of serum proteins in hyperacute lesions (Grundke-Iqbal et al. 1980). During the following remission there is some perivascular accumulation of IgG but not of fibrinogen. It is at present not resolved to what extent perivascular IgG in this stage of the disease is derived from the circulation or locally produced in perivenous plasma cells. With the onset of a relapse of the disease in the chronic stage, some perivascular accumulation of IgG and fibrin is noted which is, however, much less pronounced compared with that in the acute disease episode and restricted to the demyelinating plaques. In later stages of the disease in animals with inactive lesions in the CNS, some perivascular accumulation of immunoglobulins is found. Blood-brain barrier leakage for complement and fibrinogen was absent (Grundke-Iqbal et al. 1980). Tracer studies with horseradish peroxidase (HRP) have been performed in chronic relapsing EAE (Kristensson and Wisniewski 1977) and revealed increased vascular permeability in active as well as inactive lesions. However, many questions regarding the restoration of BBB function with chronicity of the disease and regarding the distribution of leaking vessels in the CNS have remained unresolved.

In our own studies peroxidase leakage was found in vessels of *actively demyelinating lesions* (Figs. 4, 5). In active plaques generally all vessels including arterioles, capillaries, venoles, and veins showed increased permeability, and leaking vessels could be traced for some distance into the surrounding apparently normal white matter. Increased BBB permeability was either due to enhanced transendothelial vesicular transport or to penetration of the tracer through the interendothelial extracellular space, in areas where inflammatory cells passed the endothelial lining. Within the lesions HRP was found in the extracellular space between denuded axons or intracellularly in perivascular connective tissue cells, in phagocytes and in astrocytes (Fig. 6a, b).

The vascular permeability in *inactive lesions* was variable and mainly depended upon the presence or absence of inflammatory infiltrates in the vessel walls (Fig. 4d, e). When persistent perivenous inflammation was noted together with passage of inflammatory cells through the endothelial lining, extensive perivascular accumulation of the intravenously injected tracer was found. (Figs. 4d, e, 5e, f). However, in vessels with cuffs of inflammatory cells which did not infiltrate the vascular wall, the permeability was normal or only mildly increased. Similarly in old inactive or repaired lesions a minor increase of BBB permeability was noted in the absence of inflammatory infiltrates characterized by perivascular phagocytes containing HRP reaction product (Fig. 7).

In the meninges the blood-CSF barrier was damaged in chronic relapsing EAE in focal areas corresponding to the surface extension of actively demyelinating lesions in the underlying spinal cord parenchyma (Fig. 4a, c). In the absence of actively demyelinating lesions HRP leakage was found in segments of meningeal veins which showed extensive inflammatory infiltration of the vascular wall (Fig. 8). In other segments of the same vessels, however, which were surrounded by inflammatory cells without infiltration of the walls, only a few HRP product-containing phagocytes were found (Fig. 8).

Fig. 4 a–e. Blood-brain barrier damage in chronic EAE; Hartley guinea pig 90 dps with severe chronic ▷ progressive disease; injection of horseradish peroxidase into the circulation. **a** Leptomeninges of the thoracic and lumbar spinal cord. Focal blood-brain barrier leakage in areas covering the surface of active spinal cord lesion. Isolated meninges. Peroxidase reaction, x 3. **b** Cross section of the spinal cord with peroxidase leakage in active plaques. Cryostat section, x 15. **c** Detail of **a**. Focal blood-brain barrier leakage in the meninges. x 40. **d, e** Centrum semiovale and fornix lesion showing variable peroxidase leakage *(arrows)*. Cryostat section, x 20

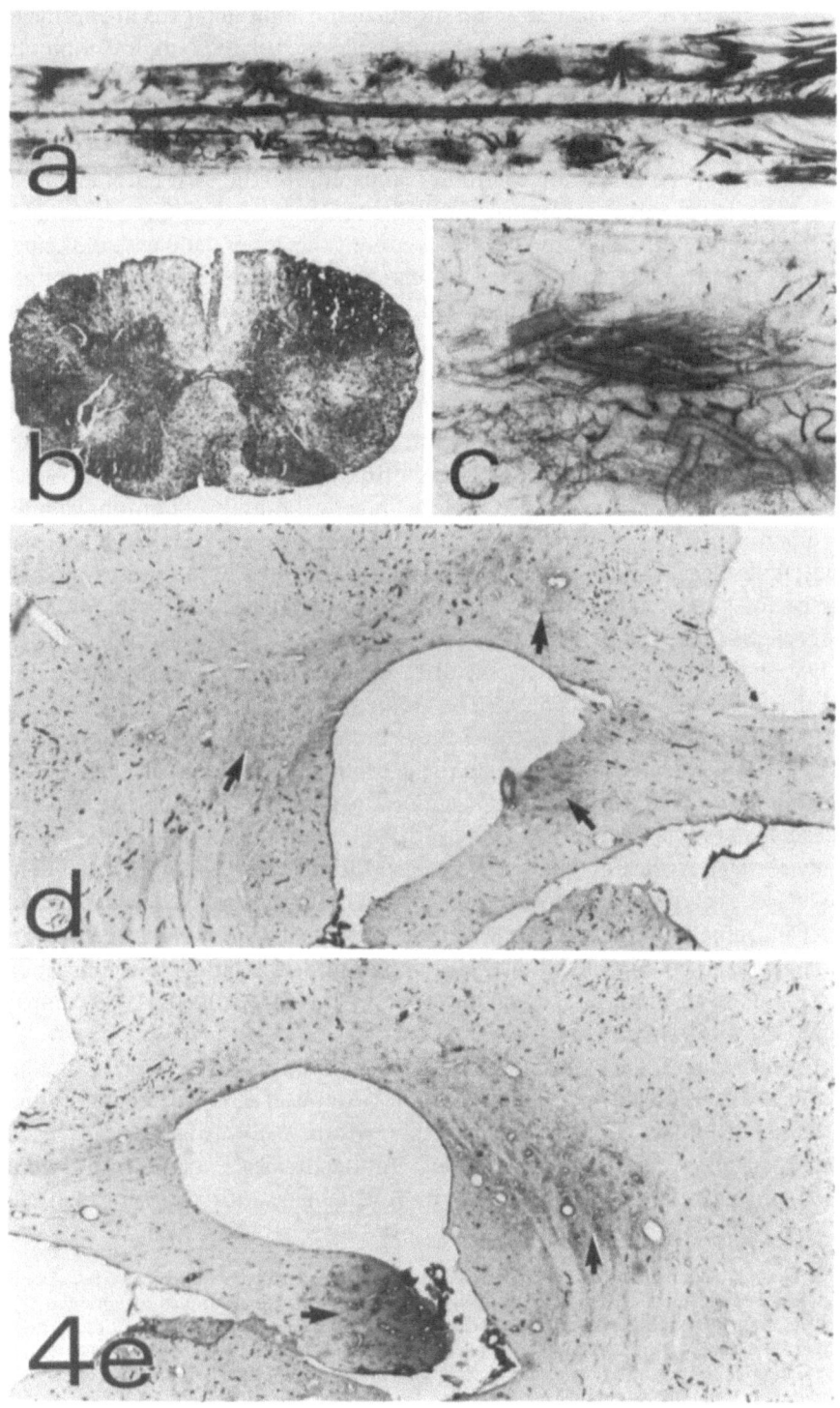

As expected HRP leakage into the stroma of the choroid plexus in chronic relapsing EAE occurred in the presence as well as absence of inflammatory infiltrates (Fig. 7c).

The number of vascular segments with increased permeability for HRP decreased with chronicity of the disease. This may be explained by the lower incidence of active lesions in the late chronic compared with the early chronic stage of the disease. In spite of the presence of BBB damage in the periplaque white matter in EAE lesions, it must be stressed that there was no general increase of the permeability of cerebral and meningeal vessels. No BBB leakage was noted in unaffected gray and white matter of the CNS, with the exception of small zones surrounding the demyelinating plaques.

These histochemical studies dealing with the distribution of endogenous serum proteins and artificial tracers in EAE lesions are valuable with regard to the localization and structural correlates of BBB damage. They are, however, of limited value in the quantitative determination of BBB dysfunction. Quantitative aspects of BBB damage and repair in EAE can be gained by the study of immunoglobulin and albumin concentration in the CNS tissue of normal and chronic EAE animals in different stages of the disease (Mehta et al. 1980, 1981). These studies revealed a massive influx of albumen and IgG into the CNS before the onset and during the acute stage of the disease (8–20 dps).

During the late stages of the acute disease episode and in the following remission the albumen levels decreased. They remained elevated, however, compared with control animals in the majority of the animals during the whole chronic stage of the disease. This indicates that with the exception of a few animals the BBB was impaired up to 250 days after sensitization. The albumen levels in the brain extracts in the chronic stage of EAE were variable from animal to animal and did not clearly correlate with different disease stages (clinical exacerbation or remission). The IgG levels in the brain and especially the IgG/albumen ratio were increased in nearly all animals sampled later than 30 days after sensitization. This, together with the presence of an oligoclonal distribution of immunoglobulins in the brain extracts, suggests an intrathecal immunoglobulin synthesis within the CNS compartment (Mehta et al. 1981).

A special aspect of these studies was that the immunohistochemical (Grundke-Iqbal et al. 1980) and immunochemical studies (Mehta et al. 1981) were performed on the same animals, thus allowing a direct comparison of histochemically visualized leakage in cerebral vessels with the immunochemical data. Both studies revealed similar results regarding the massive BBB damage during the acute episode,

---

Fig. 5 a–f. Blood-brain barrier leakage in different stages of plaque development in chronic EAE in gui- ▷
nea pigs; same animals as Fig. 4. **a, b** Border of an active plaque with extensive inflammation, active demyelination, and peroxidase leakage. **a** Toluidine blue, **b** unstained adjacent section, x 345. **c, d** Actively demyelinating lesion with massive inflammation and peroxidase leakage. **c** Toluidine blue, **d** unstained adjacent section, x 345. **e, f** Inactive lesion with persistent prevenous inflammation and blood-brain barrier leakage. **e** Toluidine blue, **f** unstained adjacent section, x 345

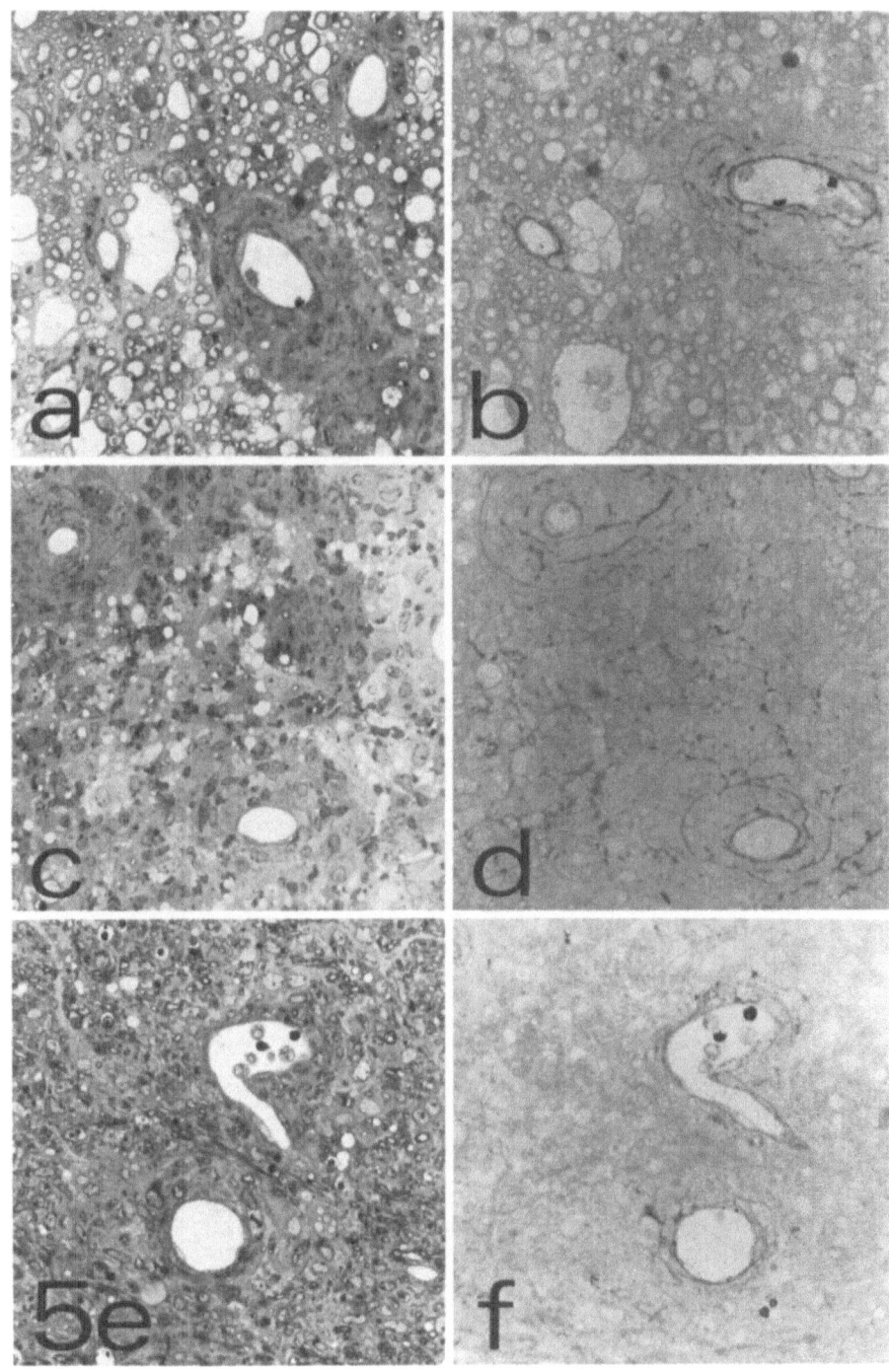

27

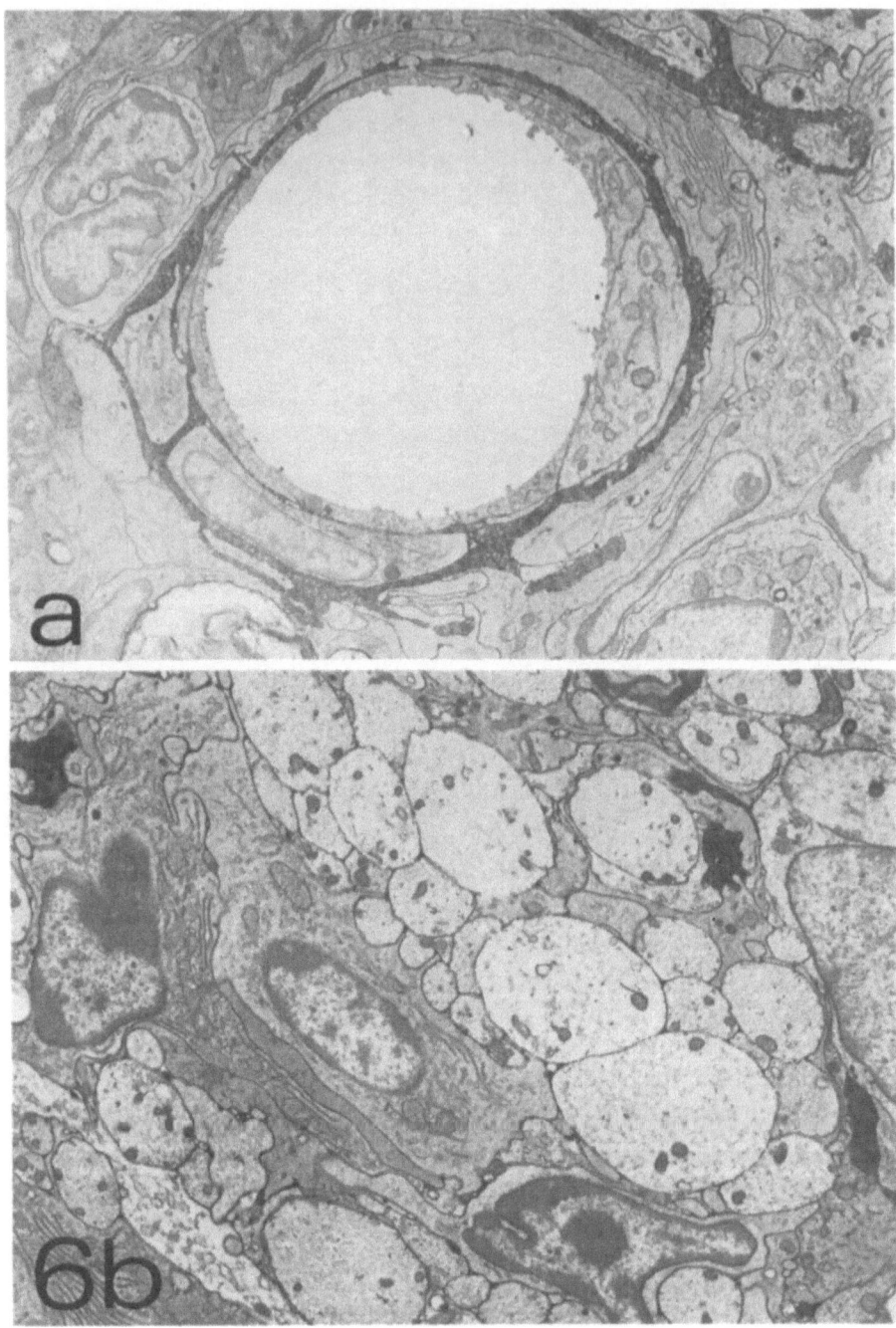

Fig. 6 a, b. Blood-brain barrier leakage in chronic EAE; same animal as in Fig. 4. **a** Small vein in an actively demyelinating lesion with severe inflammatory changes and peroxidase leakage. EM, × 3500. **b** Adjacent area to **a**; recent demyelination with peroxidase reaction product between denuded axons and inflammatory cells. EM, × 8000

28

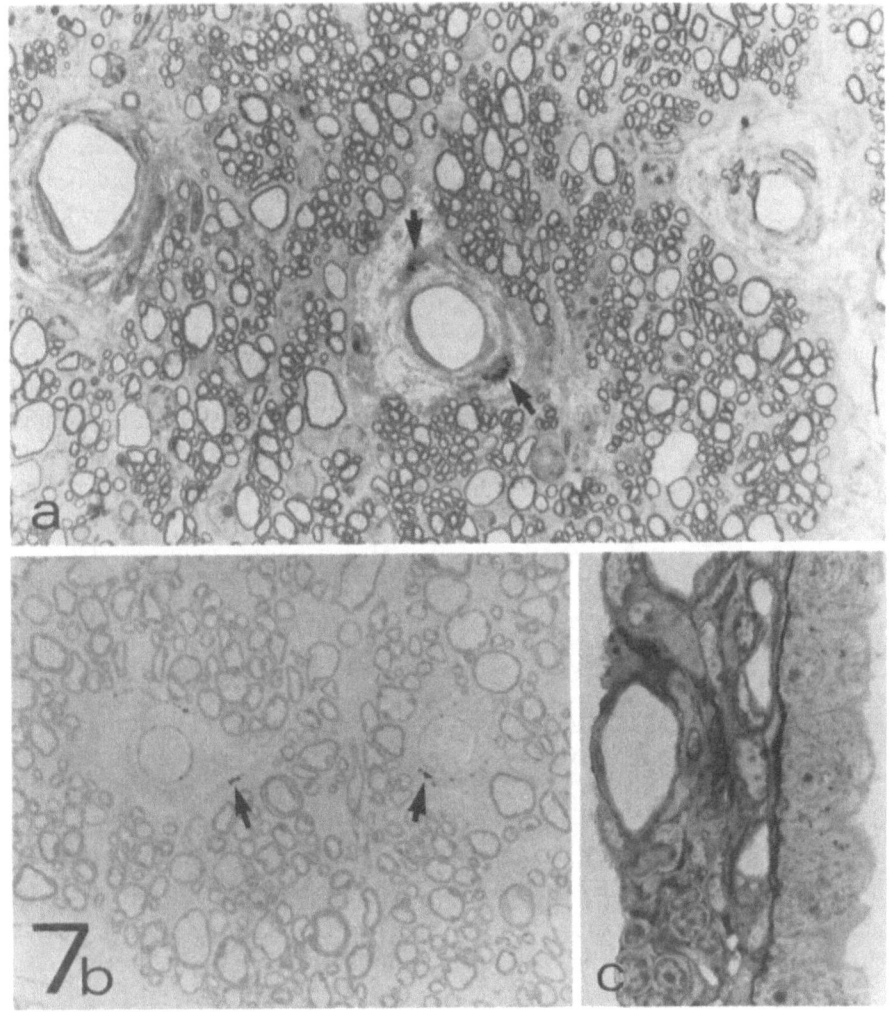

Fig. 7 a–c. Blood-brain barrier in inactive lesions; Hartley guinea pig (120 dps) with chronic relapsing EAE in remission. **a, b** Remyelinated plaque in the spinal cord with extensive capillary fibrosis. Proxidase accumulaltion in a few perivascular phagocytes *(arrows)* only. **a** Toluidine blue x 1000, **b** adjacent unstained section, x 900 **c** Choroid plexus of the same animal with some inflammation and extensive accumulation of peroxidase in the plexus stroma. Toluidine blue, x 1000

the persistent low-grade BBB damage in the chronic stage, and the presence of numerous immunoglobulin-containing plasma cells in the meninges and CNS tissue responsible for the intrathecal IgG synthesis. However, the more pronounced BBB leakage in active lesions during the first relapse of the disease shown by immunohistochemistry was not reflected by an increase of albumen in the CNS extracts which exceeded that found during inactive phases of the disease. Thus a focal BBB leakage restricted to few lesions in the CNS does not seem to affect the whole barrier in a way that it is detected by the relatively crude immunochemical techniques using pooled CNS tissue from the affected animal.

In summary, in chronic relapsing EAE several stages of the disease may be distinguished on the basis of BBB permeability. The acute stage (10–20 dps) is characterized by massive BBB damage and little or no intrathecal IgG synthesis. During the following subacute and chronic disease BBB damage is mild or moderate with increasing intrathecal IgG synthesis by plasma cells in the inflammatory infiltrates. In active lesions BBB damage is more pronounced than in inactive plaques, although less severe than in the acute stage of the disease. The partial repair of the BBB together with the presence of intrathecally synthesized IgG indicates that the immunoreaction in the chronic stage of EAE is at least partially compartmentalized in the CNS.

4.3.5 Implications of Blood-Brain Barrier Permeability on the Distribution of EAE Lesions Within the CNS

The transport of proteins through the endothelia of cerebral vessels which is present already under physiological conditions may play an important role in the induction of initial EAE lesions. Such "physiological leakage" of the BBB allows the contact between CNS antigens and the cellular and humoral immune response in sensitized animals. The presence of initial inflammatory infiltrates in meningeal vascular segments which show the highest permeability of proteins injected into the CSF (Lassmann et al., unpublished) supports this view. Furthermore, the high frequency of lesions in the anterior root entry zone in chronic relapsing EAE may be explained by a similar mechanism of increased BBB permeability (Kristensson et al. 1976). Other areas of the brain with increased BBB permeability like the area postrema and the basal hypothalamus are only rarely the target of lesions in EAE.

Fig. 8 a–e. Blood-brain barrier leakage into the meninges in the late chronic stage of chronic relasing EAE ▷ in remission. a Focal blood-brain barrier leakage in the dorsal meningeal vein. Isolated meninges, x 10. b Longitudinal section through the dorsal vein, illustrated in a (area marked by *arrow* in a); focal inflammatory infiltration of the vessel wall. Toluidine blue, x 30. c Detail of b (indicated by *arrow c*), normal vessel wall without peroxidase leakage. Toluidine blue, x 790. d, e Detail of b (indicated by *arrow d*); massive infiltration of the vessel wall by inflammatory cells and extensive peroxidase leakage. d Toluidine blue, x 985, e EM, x 3960

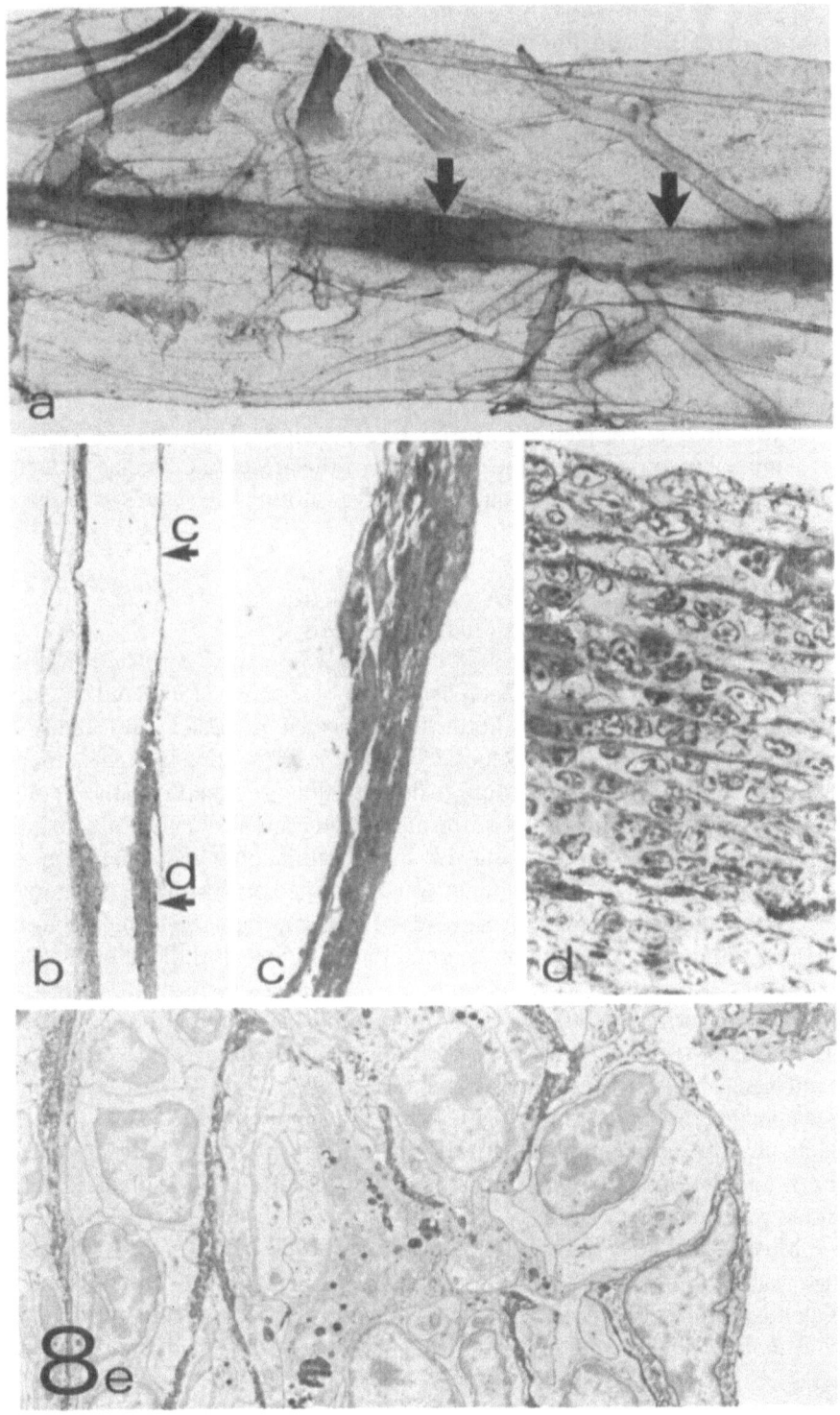

31

These regions of the brain, however, have only a low density of myelin, which may explain the infrequent localization of the lesions.

Levine (1970) described that areas which were previously affected in EAE were protected from further EAE lesions. This observation was explained by the concept of "vascular blockade" in the formation of EAE lesions. On the basis of our results in chronic relapsing EAE the concept of vascular blockade seems to be applicable for old, eventually repaired lesions but not for chronic progressive lesions. A vascular blockade is surprising in EAE as many old lesions still show increased permeability for serum proteins compared with normal cerebral vessels. However, it

cessarily behave similarly to charged proteins like myelin basic protein. Artificially cationized peroxidase, a protein with an isoelectric point like myelin basic protein, has a high affinity to collagen (Kitz et al., in preparation). Thus cationic proteins may be impeded from reaching the circulation by the presence of thick perivascular cuffs of collagen which are frequently observed around the vessels in repaired lesions.

4.3.6 The Blood-Brain Barrier in Multiple Sclerosis

Direct tracer studies in MS have been performed by Broman (1964) and by Gonsette and Andre-Basilaux (1965). Both studies showed increased permeability of blood vessels in demyelinated plaques. Control cases consisting of brain tumors, strokes, abscesses, edema, and some toxic conditions revealed negative results (Broman 1964). These findings are surprising as especially strokes, edema, and tumors should be accompanied by massive BBB dysfunction. One explanation for this discrepancy is that the experiments were performed on postmortem material, which excluded the determination of active transport mechanisms through the endothelia. Furthermore, the interpretation of these findings is difficult because of possible autolytic damage to vessel walls.

Immunohistochemical tracing of serum proteins has been performed by several authors in MS tissue (Frick 1969; Simpson et al. 1969; Lumsden 1971; Vandvik and Reske-Nielsen 1972; Tavolato 1975; Esiri 1977). Most of these studies focused upon the distribution and origin of immunoglobulins in MS lesions. Immunoglobulins were found intracellularly in inflammatory infiltrates (Lumsden 1971; Vandvik and Reske-Nielsen 1972; Esiri 1977; Mussini et al. 1977; Auff and Budka 1980) and in astrocytes (Dubois-Dalq et al. 1975; Prineas and Raine 1976; Esiri 1977; Mussini et al. 1977) as well as in the periphery especially of actively demyelinating plaques (Simpson et al. 1969; Lumsden 1971). The study of immunoglobulins alone, however, is only of limited value for determination of BBB dysfunction as it cannot be decided whether these proteins are synthesized locally or derived from the circulation. Albumen leakage in MS plaques can be regarded as a more accurate indicator of BBB damage as this protein is exclusively synthesized in the liver (Frick and Scheid-Seydel 1958; Cutler et al. 1967; Hochwald 1970). Some albumen leakage was found in old demyelinated plaques of chronic MS, but not in actively demyelinating lesions (Tavolato 1975). Albumen uptake together with IgG was observed in astrocytes, axons, and neurons in MS as well as in many other neurological diseases (Auff and Budka 1980).

Neuroradiological studies of MS patients with the CT scanner in general showed areas of decreased density corresponding to the plaque extensions (Gyldensted 1976). In acute MS, however, cranial computed tomography revealed contrast enhanced lesions (Aita et al. 1978; Wüthrich 1980), thus indicating some BBB damage.

Immunoglobulin concentration in the CSF and brain extracts of MS patients are increased together with the appearance of oligoclonal bands of immunoglobulins in 75%–88% of the investigated cases. Increased albumen levels as an indicator for BBB damage were found in 20%–30% (Link and Tibbling 1977; Eickhoff et al. 1977; Tourtellotte and Ma 1978; Tourtellotte 1970). No clear-cut correlation between the clinical stage of MS (active versus inactive) and BBB function were found (Eichhoff et al. 1977). These data indicate that the BBB is normal in more than 70% of the chronic MS cases. On the basis of our data in chronic relapsing EAE, however, the leakage of serum proteins in one or a few active focal lesions is not necessarily reflected in an overall change of BBB function in the CSF or brain extracts. On the contrary large active lesions in silent regions of the brain may reflect BBB damage in the CSF in cases with clinically remitting disease.

In summary, the data regarding BBB function in MS are conflicting and even contradictory. Nevertheless it seems to be possible to extrapolate that in cases with many active lesions, especially in acute MS, the BBB is more damaged than with typical chronic cases.

4.4 Demyelination and Myelin Degradation

The most characteristic event in the pathology of chronic relapsing EAE and multiple sclerosis is the selective destruction of myelin with relative sparing of axons, nerve cells, and other constituents of the CNS. Demyelination is restricted to the segments of the myelin sheaths, which are located within the lesions, whereas proximal and distal segments of the same neuron are unaffected. The identification of initial structural alterations of myelin sheaths and their supporting cells during active demyelination will help to understand the pathogenetic events responsible for the formation of inflammatory demyelinating lesion in EAE and MS.

Many attempts have been made in MS to identify the structural changes of myelin which may precede or occur during demyelination (Perier and Gregoire 1965; Prineas 1975; Sluga 1969; Gonatas 1970; Lumsden 1970; Prineas and Raine

1976; Prineas and Connell 1978; Kirk 1979). These studies, however, were faced with difficulties since there is considerable controversy regarding the time course of events in demyelinating lesions and the identification of actively demyelinating plaques. Thus, a sequential study of the formation of inflammatory demyelinating lesions in an experimental model will serve some framework in which the individual structural changes in MS lesions may be positioned according to their temporal relation. In chronic relapsing EAE such a sequential study is possible when several precautions are considered (Lassmann and Wisniewski 1978):

– Only spinal cord lesions can be used for this purpose. Brain lesions in guinea pigs are usually clinically silent and make clinicopathological correlation impossible.
– Animals must manifest clinically a clear-cut relapsing disease pattern with sudden onset of the first relapse of the disease. In such a disease course healthy animals develop complete paraparesis of hind legs within few hours of onset of the relapse.
– The relapse must be short lasting with improvement of the clinical status a few days after onset of the exacerbation of the disease.

4.4.1 Initial Stages of Demyelination in EAE

The initial step in plaque formation in chronic relapsing EAE, which can be found during the first hours after onset of a relapse, is the invasion of large mononuclear cells from the perivenous space into the CNS tissue. Simultaneously in these areas myelin is fragmented, and myelin sheaths and myelin fragments are stained by the Marchi reaction. Small droplets of myelin are incorporated in phagocytes. These so-called myelin balls (Seitelberger 1960) still have the same staining properties as normal myelin, with the exception of the Marchi and OTAN reaction.

In electron microscopy several different patterns of myelin destruction may be found in this stage of plaque formation:

1. The direct attack of phagocytes on the myelin sheath: This pattern, designed as "myelin stripping," is initiated by an intimate contact of the macrophage cell membrane with the myelin sheath followed by separation and rupture of myelin lamellae and the invasion of macrophage cell processes or whole cells between individual lamellae of the myelin sheaths (Lampert 1965; Lampert and Kies 1967; Wisniewski et al. 1969). Although this process of myelin destruction may start at any point of the internode (Lampert 1965), the paranodal regions of the sheath are more frequently affected (Madrid and Wisniewski 1978). Simultaneously with the invasion of macrophages into the myelin sheaths, profound changes of the myelin segment along the whole internode may take place, with splitting of myelin lamellae and disintegration of the sheaths (Madrid and Wisniewski 1978). Myelin fragments are ingested by phagocytes.

2. Another pattern of demyelination can be found in EAE lesions, most pronounced in certain models of hyperacute EAE, but also in models of ordinary or

chronic EAE. In this type, which is generally accompanied by extensive intra- and extramyelinic edema, a direct involvement of phagocytes is rarely observed. The myelin sheath shows splitting of individual lamellae, sometimes leading to massive ballooning of the sheaths. Other myelin segments are uniformly transformed into small single- or multilayered lipid vesicles, surrounding the axon as a foamy network. This pattern of demyelination is described as "vesicular transformation" or "vesicular disruption of myelin" (Lampert 1965, 1967; Dal Canto et al. 1975). In general in most EAE models both types of demyelination can be found simultaneously (Lampert 1965; Lampert and Kies 1967), in variable quantitative proportions, however. It is thus not clear at the present time whether vesicular disruption of myelin is just a more severe variant of the same pathogenetic process which leads to myelin stripping. There is, however, some indirect evidence that vesicular disruption of myelin is indeed due to a different pathogenetic type of myelin destruction. This type of demyelination in chronic EAE may be found predominantly in models which are characterized by a weak perivascular macrophage response and by extensive degradation of myelin in local (astroglia or oligodendroglia) cells. Furthermore, vesicular disruption of myelin is the dominant pattern of demyelination induced by EAE sera injected into the cerebrospinal fluid (Lassmann et al. 1981c) or into peripheral nerves (Saida et al. 1979c), models in which the macrophage response is much less intense than in classical EAE (Saida et al. 1979c; Lassmann et al. 1981c).

It is now well established that myelin stripping and vesicular disruption of myelin are very characteristic patterns of demyelination in EAE. This, however, does not exclude that other less characteristic changes of myelin may precede demyelination. In this connection it is interesting that even in most rapidly demyelinating lesions in chronic relapsing EAE structural changes resembling myelin stripping or vesicular disruption of myelin are rare. Patterns of demyelination, however, which have no similarly unique structural appearance, cannot be differentiated clearly from fixation artifacts and thus cannot be identified as initial stages of demyelination.

4.4.2 Myelin Degradation and Removal of Debris in EAE

The time course and sequence of myelin destruction can be easily followed in chronic relapsing EAE. Myelin degradation is performed in a similar way to in experimental models of secondary myelin destruction or in human inflammatory demyelinating diseases (Seitelberger 1960; Lampert and Cressmann 1966; Lassmann et al. 1978a). Light microscopically an initial stage of physical myelin disintegration (Seitelberger 1960), which is expressed mainly by swelling and vesicle formation within the myelin sheath, is followed by ingestion of small lipid droplets ("myelin balls"; Seitelberger 1960) into phagocytes. The myelin balls still retain the staining characteristics of normal myelin with routine lipid stains (Seitelberger 1960; Hallpike and Adams 1969; Hallpike et al. 1970) are positive in the Marchi or OTAN method and seem to be depleted from some of the myelin proteins, especially myelin basic protein (Hallpike and Adams 1969). Ultrastructurally these inclusions are osmiophilic and composed of uniformly layered lipid membranes with a periodicity of 40–50 A (Lassmann et al. 1978a, b; Lassmann and Wisniewski 1979c). It is questionable whether the first stage of physical disintegration of myelin always represents an initial stage of myelin destruction. Secondary myelin changes due to edema or unspecific inflammatory mediators and fixation artifacts cannot be exluded, as these changes are sometimes also found around otherwise inactive lesions. The presence of myelin balls (Luxol fast blue positive degradation products) can be demonstrated at least 10–14 days after onset of demyelination, or sometimes even longer when demyelination is progressing. About 10 days after onset of a clear-cut clinical relapse first PAS-positive or sudanophilic degradation products (Lassmann and Wisniewski 1979c) are noted in the lesions. These myelin degradation products may then be found in the plaques for variable time intervals as long as several weeks. The amount of sudanophilic degradation products is variable in different animal species. Marked accumulation of sudanophilic lipids within gitter cells are found in EAE lesions in monkeys (Roizin 1949; Seitelberger 1960) whereas in small rodents like guinea pigs and rats the sudanophilic stage of myelin degradation is sparse or absent (Lassmann and Wisniewski 1979c).

An interesting feature of myelin degradation in chronic relapsing EAE in guinea pigs is the prevalence of PAS-positive degradation products during the stage of chemical degradation of myelin lipids (Lassmann and Wisniewski 1979c). This ultrastructurally pleomorphic debris is present quantitatively in much higher amounts than with conditions where myelin is destroyed secondarily (e.g., Wallerian degeneration or ischemic necrosis). Although the significance of this finding in the pathogenesis of the disease is not yet defined, there are several possible explanations for this observation. Myelin degradation and debris removal may take a slower course in EAE compared with ischemic or traumatic CNS injury. Therefore the amount of liberated cholesterin esters and triglycerides may be smaller at any given time during degradation and thus allow the cells to reutilize or further degrade the sudanophilic material. Such an event will result in a relative increase in other degradation products. Alternatively, autoimmune demyelination may result in accumulation of lipid debris dressed with, or altered by, antibodies or inflammatory mediators, which are then difficult to degrade and thus accumulate in the degrading cells.

The clearance of plaques from debris-containing phagocytes follows different time courses, depending on the localization of the lesion, on the animal species, and especially on the involvement of local cells in the degradation of myelin. In spinal cord lesions immediately beneath the meninges, debris removal may be very rapid, even in large plaques, and in some animals is completed as soon as 14 days after plaque formation. When lesions are located in the depth of the white matter or especially when local cells are involved in the removal of myelin, debris-containing phagocytes are present in the plaques for at least several weeks (Lassmann et al. 1980b).

It is generally believed that in EAE myelin degradation is performed mainly in hematogenous macrophages (Kosunen et al. 1963; Lampert and Carpenter 1965; Smith and Waksman 1969). This view is based upon the observations that perivenous monocytes invade the lesions during the stage of active demyelination, are then directly involved in demyelination with myelin stripping and uptake of debris, and finally leave the parenchyma by accumulation in perivenous or pericapillary spaces. Autoradiographic and electron microscopic studies have also shown that the majority of phagocytes in acute EAE are derived from the circulation (Kosunen et al. 1963; Bubis and Luse 1964; Lampert and Carpenter 1965) although local microglia and pericytes seem to play an additional role in removal of debris in inflammatory conditions of the CNS (Oehmichen et al. 1973) (Figs. 10, 11). When demyelination is induced by EAE sera in tissue culture no hematogenous macrophages are available, and degradation of debris is thus performed exclusively in local cells including astrocytes (Raine and Bornstein 1970a). A similar picture may be noted when demyelinated plaques are investigated which occur in animal species with a relatively weak macrophage response in the initial stage of lesion formation (Lassmann et al. 1980b). In chronic EAE lesions in Sprague Dawley rats a considerable proportion of debris is taken up and digested in astrocytes (Fig. 9), even in cells which can be identified as oligodendrocytes in remyelinating lesions (Figs. 9, 12). Involvement of oligodendrocytes in degradation of myelin has been previously noted in Wallerian degeneration (Cook and Wisniewski 1973; Lassmann et al. 1978a). In EAE it is however, not possible at present, to determine whether debris-containing oligodendrocytes originate from the myelin-supporting cells directly or whether a pool of undifferentiated glia cells (Vaughn et al. 1970) first take up debris and then differentiate to mature oligodendrocytes.

4.4.3 Demyelination and Myelin Degradation in Multiple Sclerosis

In multiple sclerosis the initial structural changes leading to demyelination are still conflicting. This is due mainly to difficulties in identification of active lesions. The most frequent alterations of myelin in lesions which were believed to be active were splitting of myelin lamellae (Perier and Gregorie 1965; Suzuki et al. 1969; Gonatas 1970) and the formation of small intramyelinic vesicles (de Preux and Mair 1974; Lumsden 1970; Kirk 1979). Both changes, especially when present at low incidence, may occur as fixation artifacts and in other conditions where myelin is destroyed (Thomas and Sheldon 1964). More recently a peculiar alteration of myelin sheaths has been described and interpreted as initial stage of demyelination in MS (Prineas and Connell 1978). This alteration, called "micropinocytosis vermiformis", was characterized by engulfment of myelin lamellae in straight or curved

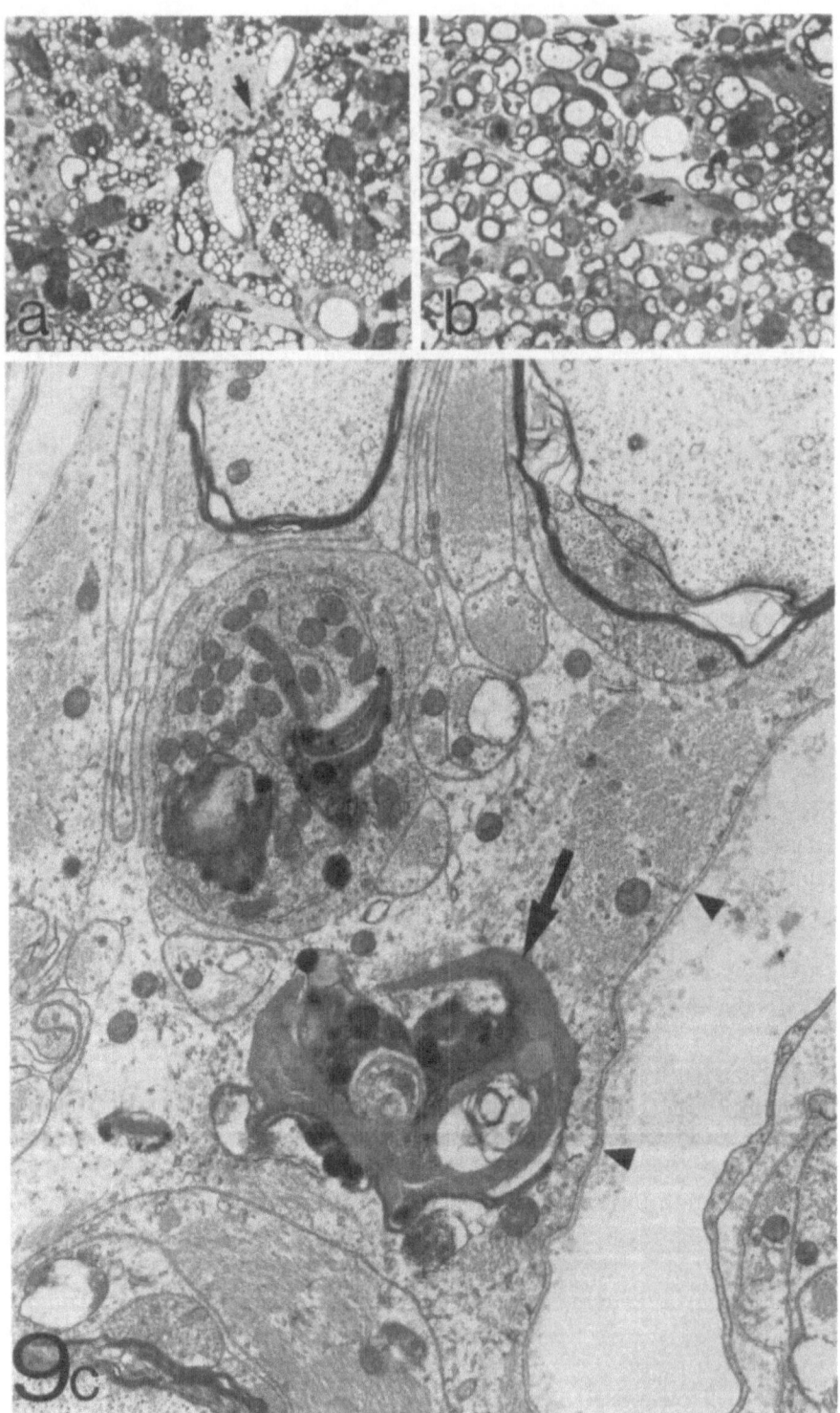

38

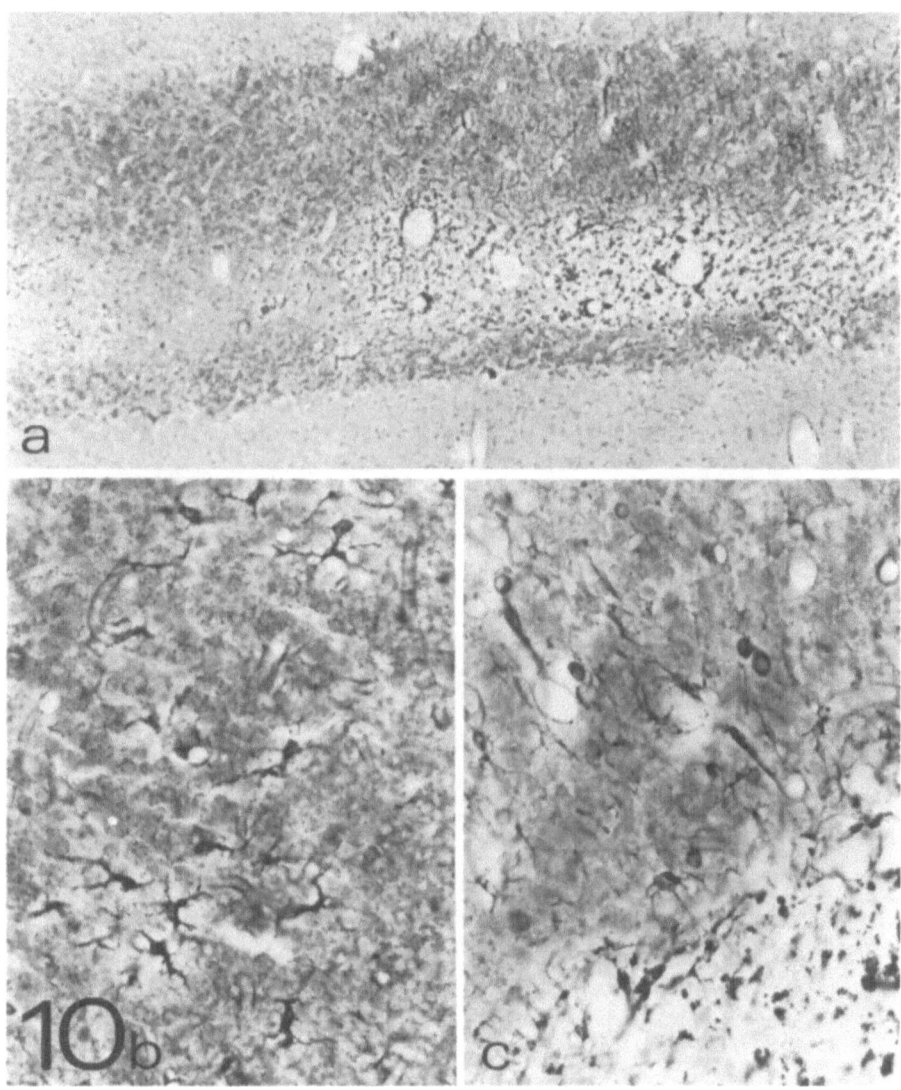

Fig. 10 a–c. Chronic EAE lesions in Sprague Dawley rats; Weil-Davenport silver impregnation for oligodendroglia and microglia; cerebellar white matter. **a** Small demyelinated lesion in the white matter with
increased silver positive cells in the plaque and in the periplaque tissue. x 80. **b** Detail of **a**; so-called activated microglia in the cerebellar cortex adjacent to the lesion. x 400. **c** "Activated microglia" and normal
oligodendrologia in the periplaque area. x 400

◁ **Fig. 9 a–c.** Chronic EAE lesions in Spraque Dewleay rats; myelin degradation in astrocytes. **a, b** Demyelinated, partially remyelinated EAE lesions; osmiophilic debris in large reactive astrocytes *(arrows)*. Toluidine blue, **a** x 700, **b** x 1000. **c** Similar lesion to in **a**; late myelin debris *(large arrow)* in an astrocytic
process of the glia limitans *(small arrows)*. EM, x 9950

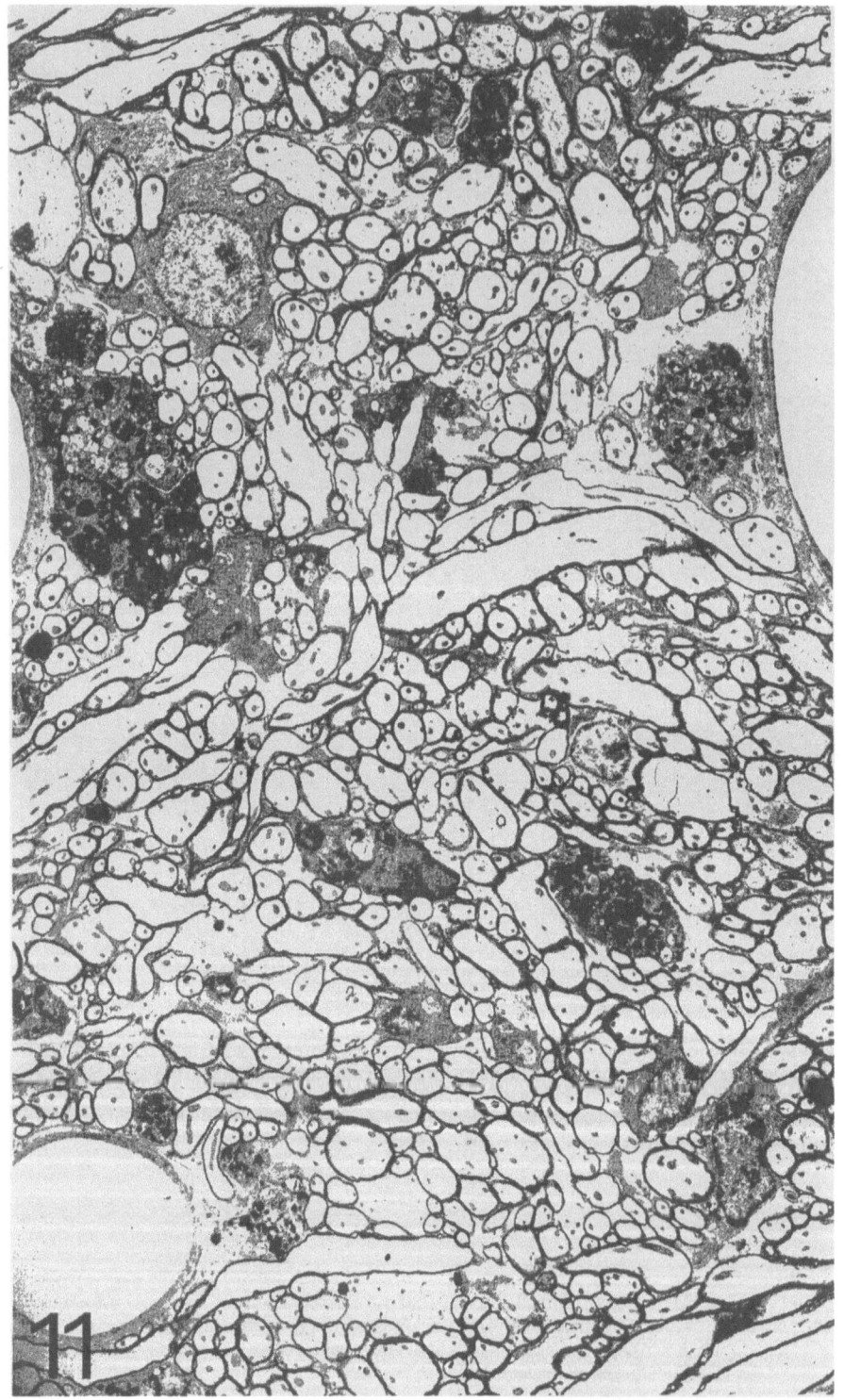

11

40

indentations of the cytoplasm of putative phagocytes. The cytoplasmic surface of the tubular indentations was surrounded by granular material similar to coated vescicles. There are, however, doubts regarding the activity of the described lesions, especially because of the lack of recent myelin degradation products. The above discussed studies have based the identification of active plaques in MS mainly on the presence of sudanophilic myelin degradation products and did not document the presence of earlier stages of myelin degradation. From histochemical evidence in MS lesions, however, it is well known that the sudanophilic stage of myelin degradation is not a marker for initial lesions (Seitelberger 1960; Lumsden 1970; Adams 1975).

Lumsden (1970) identified actively demyelinating plaques by the presence of the earliest stages of myelin debris. In this study active lesions showed pronounced edema and astroglia swelling. Myelin sheaths frequently revealed splitting of myelin lamellae, together with the formation of intramyelinic vacuoles and sometimes ballooning of myelin sheaths. In addition some myelin sheaths were transformed into small vesicles, closely resembling vesicular disruption of myelin (Lumsden 1970).

Recently we have studied the patterns of demyelination in autopsy cases of acute and chronic MS collected in our institute during the past years (Lassmann et al., in preparation). For this purpose hypercellular plaques were screened by light microscopy to localize areas with the earliest detectable myelin degradation products (myelin balls; Seitelberger 1960). Corresponding blocks of the selected areas were embedded in Epon and studied light and electron microscopically. In acute MS (Marburg's type) the most frequent initial alteration in all investigated lesions was extensive vesicular disruption of myelin (Fig. 13). This vesicular transformation either involved the whole myelin sheath or was localized in the inner or outer loops of the sheaths, especially near the node of Ranvier. In the same areas frequently invasion of phagocytes or their cell processes into the myelin sheaths was noted (Fig. 14). Intramyelinic phagocytes were predominantly localized near the node of Ranvier; their cell bodies or processes were found either between the axon and the meylin sheath or between individual myelin lamellae. In the vicinity of the phagocytes the myelin sheath was frequently ruptured, distorted, or revealed vesicular disruption. In between the completely or partially demyelinated nerve fibers numerous phagocytes were observed which contained fragments of the myelin sheaths. In addition to these characteristic myelin alterations other myelinated fibers showed assymmetrical and discontinuous thinning of myelin sheaths, especially at the nodes of Ranvier and the removal and investigation of large myelin fragments by phagocytes (Fig. 15).

◁ **Fig. 11.** Chronic EAE lesions in Sprague Dawley rats; remyelinated lesion in the cerebellar white matter; numerous microglia-like cells with debris. EM, x 2000

41

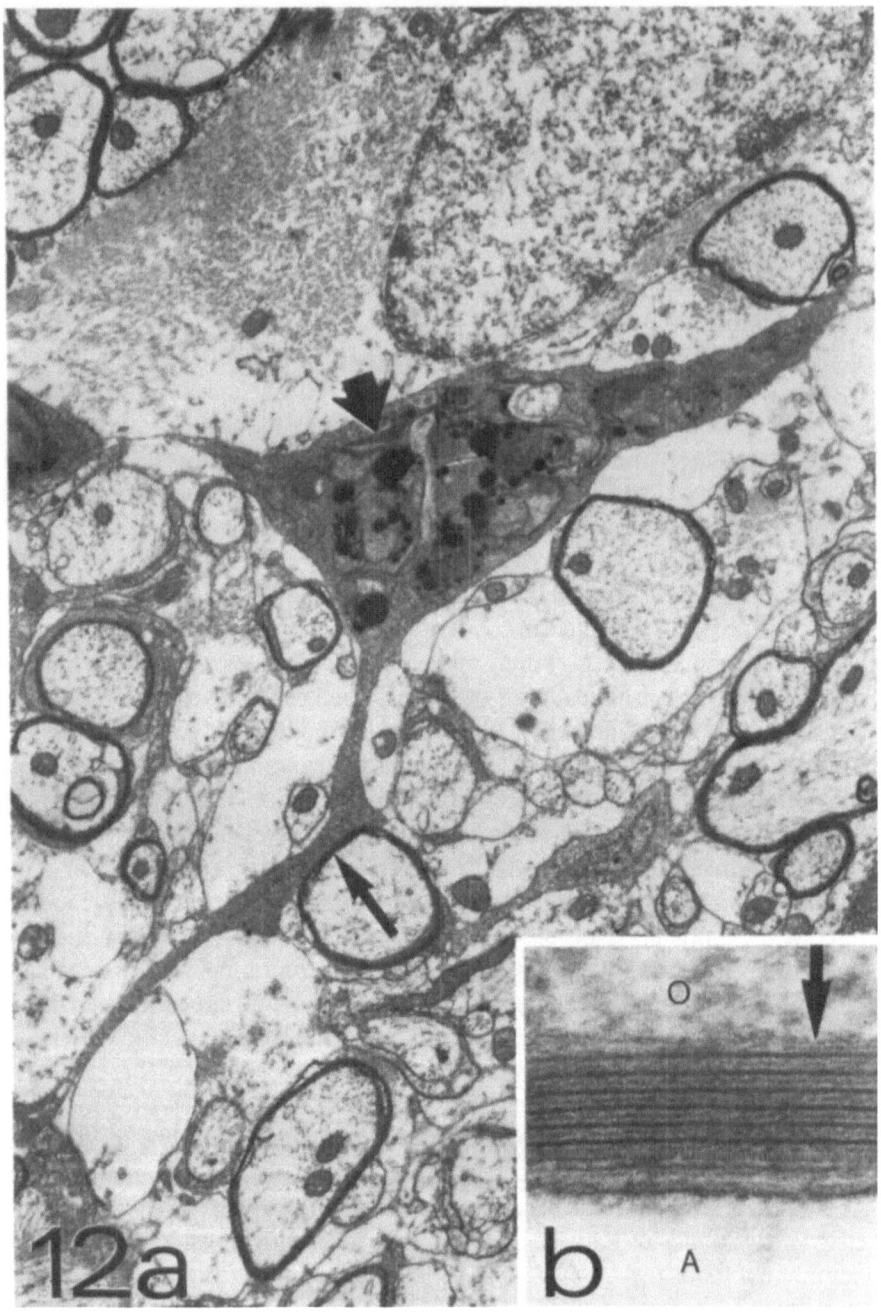

Fig. 12 a, b. Chronic EAE lesion in Sprague Dawley rat; remyelinated lesion in the cerebellar white matter; oligodendrocyte nature of some of the microglia-like cells. **a** "Microglia cell" *(large arrow)* with cellular process in close contact to newly formed myelin *(small arrow)*. EM x 8000. **b** Detail of **a** (indicated by *small arrow)*; the cell membrane of the cell process is the outermost lamella of the myelin sheath. *O,* oligodendroglia cytoplasma; *A,* axon. EM, x 170000

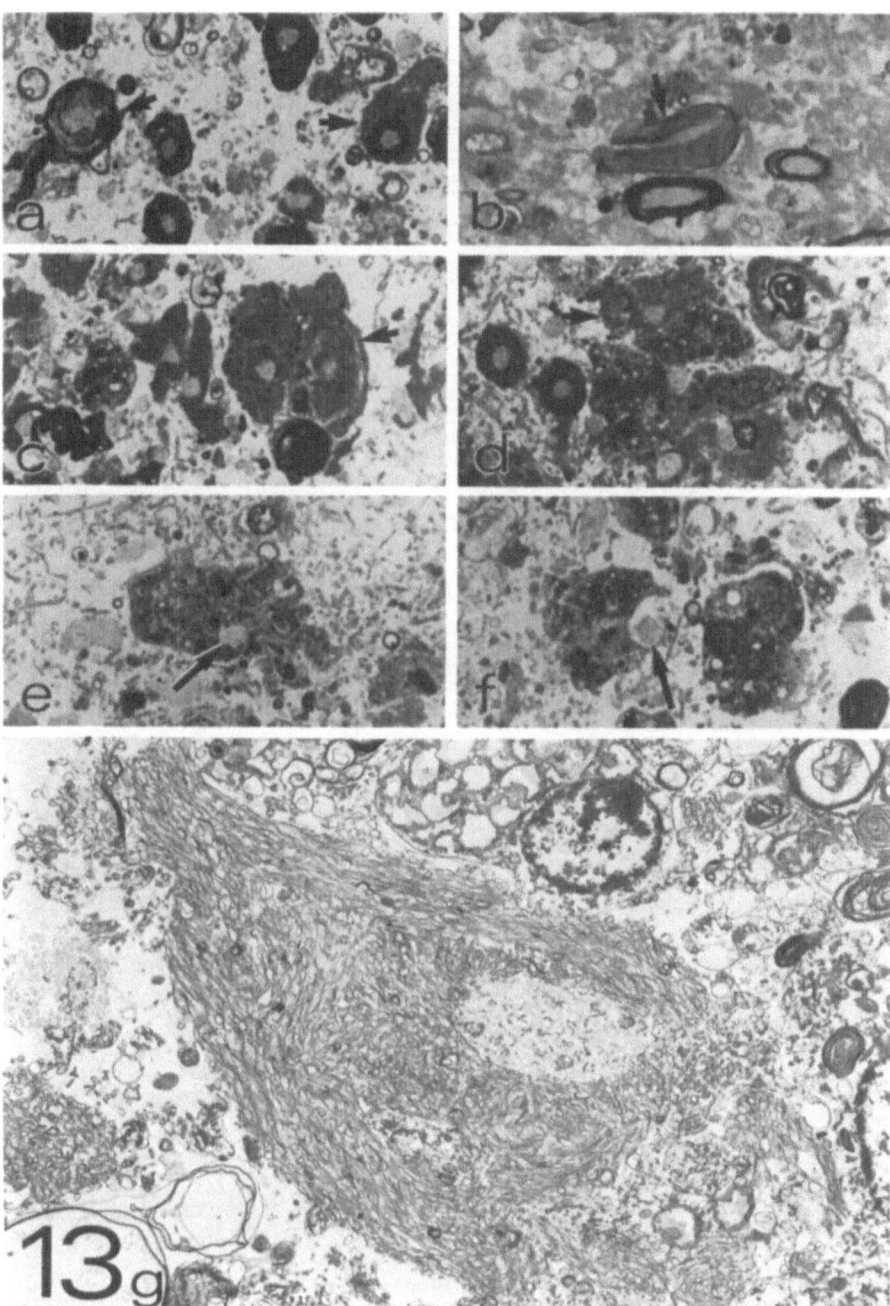

Fig. 13 a–g. Vesicular disruption of myelin in multiple sclerosis: 26-year-old female with acute MS, leading to death 12 weeks after onset of the disease (detailed clinical history and neuropathology published by Lassmann et al. 1981d); active lesion in the frontal white matter. **a–f** Different stages of vesicular disruption. Toluidine blue, x 1000. **a, b** Transformation of inner or outer parts of the myelin sheat into moderately osmiophilic homogeneous material *(arrows)*. **c, d** Complete transformation of myelin into the above-described material and the beginning of phagocytosis of the debris *(arrows)*. The axons appear as light disks in the center of the material. **e, f** Phagocytosis of the material by macrophages; axons are still visible as light disks in the center *(arrows)*. **g** Electron micrograph of **c**; the whole myelin sheath is transformed into small lipid vesicles. EM, x 3500

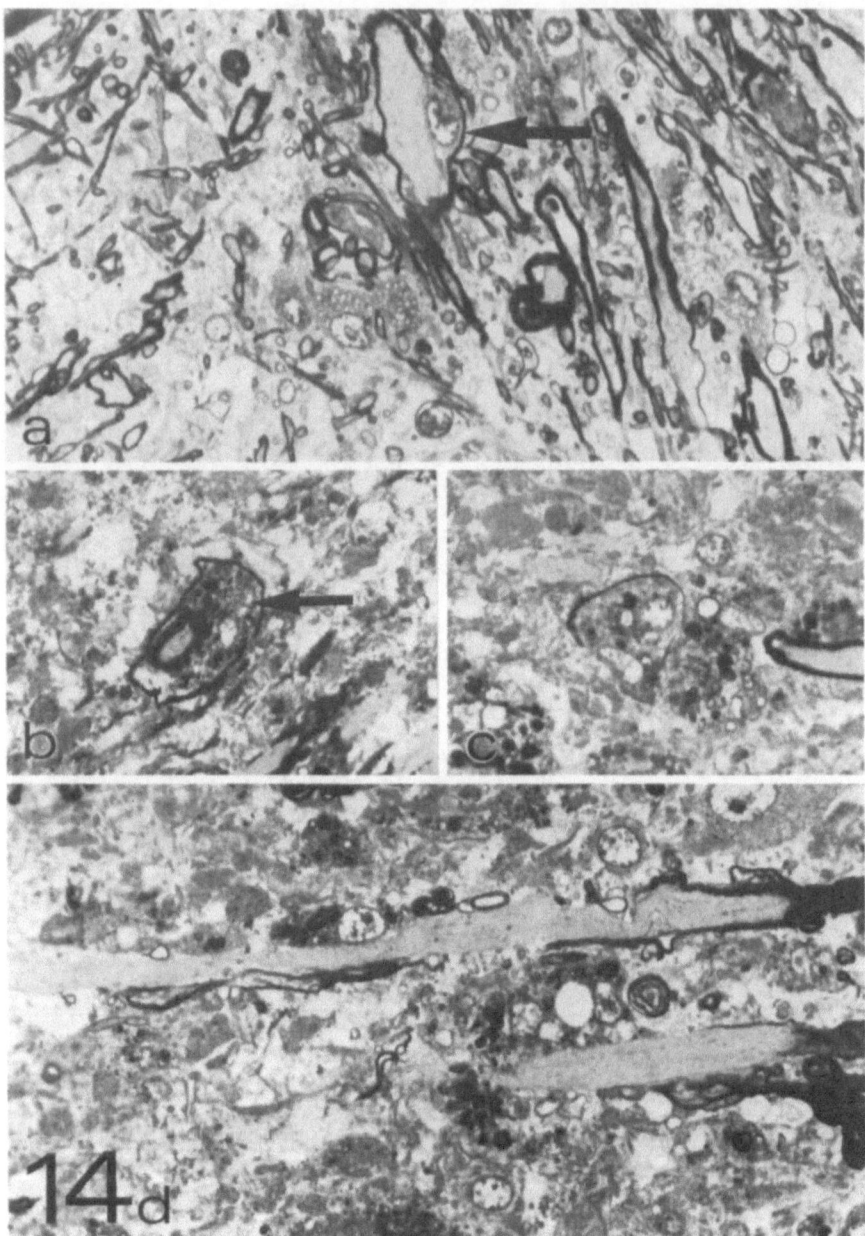

Fig. 14 a–d. Invasion of phagocytes into the myelin sheaths (myelin stripping) in acute multiple sclerosis. **a** Same lesion as described in Fig. 13; a phagocyte between the axon and the myelin sheath *(arrow)* Toluidine blue, × 1000. **b, c** 21-year-old male with subacute MS, leading to death 14 months after onset of the disease; relapsing disease course with rapid progression during the last 4 months; active lesion in the brain stem. **b** Phagocyte with debris, invaded between lamellae of the myelin sheath *(arrow)*. Toluidine blue, × 1000. **c** Phagocyte surrounded by thin myelin sheath. Toluidine blue, × 1000. **d** Active brain stem lesion in the patient described in Fig. 13; asymmetrical removal of myelin from a large axon. Toluidine blue, × 1000

44

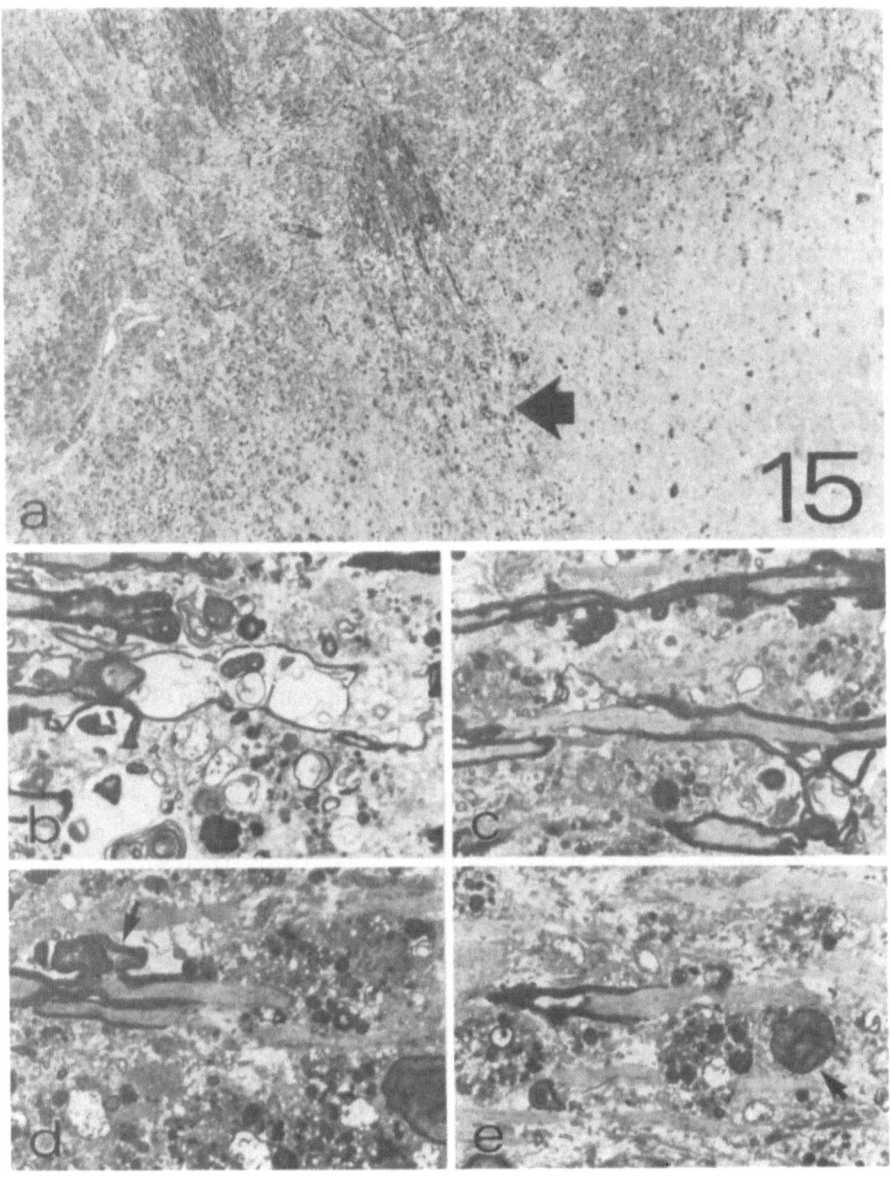

Fig. 15 a–e. Initial myelin alterations in active lesions in chronic multiple sclerosis; female with chronic relapsing MS with rapid progression, leading to death 2 years after onset of the disease; multiple large demyelinated plaques in autopsy, the majority with ongoing demyelinating activity throughout the whole brain and spinal cord. **a** Active zone in the periphery of a large demyelinated plaque in the pons. The border between the normal white matter and the plaque, with numerous phagocytes, which contain early stages of myelin debris *(arrow)*. Toluidine blue, X 100. **b–e** Details of **a**. Toluidine blue, X 1000. **b** Ballooning of myelin sheaths. **c** Asymmetrical thinning of myelin at the node of Ranvier. **d, e** Large globules of myelin either in continuity with the myelin sheath (**d** *arrow*) or internalized in phagocytes (**e** *arrow*)

Active plaques in chronic MS differed in several respects from the demyelinating lesions in acute MS. The intensity of perivenous inflammatory reaction together with the hypercellularity of actively demyelinating areas was less pronounced in chronic versus acute MS lesions. Initial stages of demyelination included some vesicular disruption of myelin, although complete vesicular transformation of the whole myelin sheath was rarely observed. Invasion of phagocytes or their processes into the myelin sheaths was rare in active lesions of chronic MS. The main structural changes of myelin consisted of intramyelinic edema with massive swelling of the sheaths, the removal and ingestion of large myelin fragments by phagocytes, widening of the node of Ranvier, and paranodal asymmetrical thinning and removal of myelin sheaths (Fig. 15).

Because of the limited material available it is at present not clear whether these differences between active lesions in acute and chronic MS are due to variations in velocity and severity of the disease process or due to dissimilarities in the pathogenetic events leading to demyelination.

Further myelin degradation in MS follows a histological, histochemical, and ultrastructural pattern similar to that found in other inflammatory demyelinating diseases of the CNS or that of diseases with secondary destruction of myelin sheaths (Seitelberger 1960; Lumsden 1970; Sluga 1979). There is, however, some indication that myelin degradation is retarded compared with diseases with secondary demyelination (Lumsden 1970). This view is based mainly upon observations regarding clinicopathological correlations, comparisons with other plaque features (gliosos, morphology of plaque edges, etc.), and upon the abundance of granular, ultrastructurally pleomorphic myelin debris. Similar to that in EAE, myelin degradation starts with a stage of physical disintegration of myelin sheaths followed by a stage of "myelin balls" (Seitelberger 1960; Lumsden 1970). Then chemical degradation of myelin lipids takes place, resulting in the appearance of sudanophilic and PAS-positive material. The exact time course of these changes is not yet defined; however, sudanophilic lipids seem to be present within the lesions up to several months after plaque formation (Lumsden 1970).

The abundance of PAS-positive, ultrastructurally pleomorphic degradation products has recently raised some attention in ultrastructural studies of MS pathology (Prineas 1975; Sluga 1979; Prineas and Wright 1978) and has been postulated as highly characteristic for early MS plaques (Prineas 1975). Similar lysosomal inclusions, however, may also be found in progressive multifocal leukoencephalopathy (Hauw and Escourolle 1977) and to a minor degree in Wallerian degradation in experimental animals (Lassmann et al. 1978a) and humans (Lassmann, unpublished). These degradation products are in addition very similar to those found in large amounts in chronic relapsing EAE (Lassmann and Wisniewski 1979c). As in the latter disease the significance of these observations in MS is still unresolved.

Myelin degradation in MS is performed in general in so-called gitter cells. Their precise origin (hematogenous or local) has so far not been clear. The perivenous and pericapillary accumulation of debris-containing cells, which, as discussed above, may be an indicator for their hematogenous origin, varies from case to case and also within different plaques in the same case. As a general rule, however, pericapillary accumulation of debris-containing phagocytes is more pronounced in acute MS than in active lesions in chronic MS. However, in both acute and chronic MS, a minor fraction of the myelin debris can also be found in typical local cells of the CNS (Marburg 1906; Sluga 1979).

In summary, the patterns of demyelination and myelin degradation are very similar in chronic EAE and multiple sclerosis, provided active lesions are identified in MS on the basis of myelin degradation products. It must be emphasized, however that the presence of vesicular disruption of myelin and myelin stripping in MS does not necessarily imply that pathogentic mechanisms similar to those in EAE are responsible for myelin damage. Myelin stripping as initial damage in demyelination may occur in EAE induced by myelin basic protein (MBP) as well as by whole CNS tissue (Lampert 1965; Lampert and Kies 1967). Furthermore, a similar pattern of myelin damage may be induced by injection of EAE sera into the CSF of normal recipient animals (Lassmann et al. 1981) or even in models of bystander demyelination (Wisniewski and Bloom 1975). Thus, several different pathogenetic mechanisms may lead to similar initial ultrastructural patterns of demyelination.

4.5 The Fate of Oligodendroglia

Oligodendrocytes are generally lost or reduced in number in chronic sclerotic lesions in multiple sclerosis and chronic EAE (McAlpine et al. 1955; Ibrahim and Adams 1963; Lumsden 1970; Synder et al. 1975a; Lassmann and Wisniewski 1979a). The interpretation of oligodendrocyte alterations is of special importance for the pathogenetic interpretation of demyelinating lesions. The presence or absence of structural changes in oligodendrocytes preceding or occurring during demyelination will answer the question of whether the disease process is primarily directed against myelin or whether demyelination follows alterations or destruction of oligodendrocytes.

4.5.1 Oligodendrocytes in EAE Lesions

In acute EAE Lampert (1965) describes the ensheathment and destruction of oligodendroglia cell processes by mononuclear cells in actively demyelinating lesions. This finding was substantiated by the study of serial sections, which established the relationship of these cell processes to myelin sheaths. In other studies degeneration of cells which were believed to be oligodendrocytes were observed in demyelinating EAE lesions (Bubis and Luse 1964; Field and Raine 1969) (Fig. 17). The significance of these observations, however, is uncertain because of difficulties in the identification of oligodendrocytes in demyelinated lesions. In normal CNS tissue oligodendrocytes are well characterized by their relationship to myelin sheaths (Peters 1968) and by their nuclear and cytoplasmic structural features (Mori and Leblond 1970) (Fig. 16). In demyelinated plaques and especially in active lesions the cellular relationship to myelin sheaths is lost. Furthermore, mononuclear cells with sometimes striking ultrastructural similarities to oligodendrocytes appear in the lesions and also may degenerate and be phagocytosed by other mononuclear cells (Lampert 1965; Lampert and Kies 1967). Thus, Lampert and Kies (1967) came to the conclusion that it is virtually impossible to identify a degenerating cell in actively demyelinating lesions as an oligodendrocyte by electron microscopy. In spite of several subsequent ultrastructural studies of acute and chronic EAE lesions (Dal Canto et al. 1975; Prineas et al. 1969; Raine et al. 1974), the problems of identification of oligodendrocytes in active lesions remain the same (Fig. 17). It must be observed, however, that degeneration of oligodendrocytes in the well-myelinated perilesional zone surrounding active plaques in EAE has not been documented.

Indirect information regarding the fate of oligodendrocytes in chronic EAE lesions may be obtained from the study of inactive or partially repaired lesions. In these lesions inflammatory cells which may be misinterpreted as oligodendrocytes have vanished and a variable degree of remyelination allows accurate identification of myelin-supporting cells. When such inactive lesions are studied, the degree of oligodendrocyte loss in chronic EAE lesions seems to be variable, depending mainly upon the time interval between sensitization and plaque formation (Lassmann et al. 1980b). In the acute, subacute, and early chronic stage of the disease (10–100 days after sensitization), cells resembling the light and electron microscopic features of oligodendrocytes can be found in high numbers in the lesions (Figs. 17, 18f, g), and remyelination may take place within 1–2 weeks after plaque formation (Lampert 1965; Lassmann et al. 1980b). On the contrary in lesions formed during the late chronic stage of the disease (100–200 dps in Hartley guinea pigs) mainly astrocytes and their processes are found between the denuded axons (Fig. 21). Cells resembling oligodendrocytes are lost or reduced in numbers (Fig. 18a-e), and remyelination is sparse and predominantly located at the lesional borders (Fig. 18a-e). Thus, whereas in acute and early chronic lesions the myelin sheath is nearly exclusively destroyed, in lesions developing during the late chronic stage oligodendrocytes are affected in addition to myelin. This indicates that with increasing time after sensitization target structures which contain even a low density of myelin antigens are more effectively destroyed. Alternatively animals with prolonged course of chronic EAE may develop additional immune responses directed not only against myelin but also against oligodendroglia antigens.

In demyelinated lesions in the cortex or in the brain stem nuclei the perineural satellite cells which at least morphologically are similar to oligodendrocytes are unaffected.

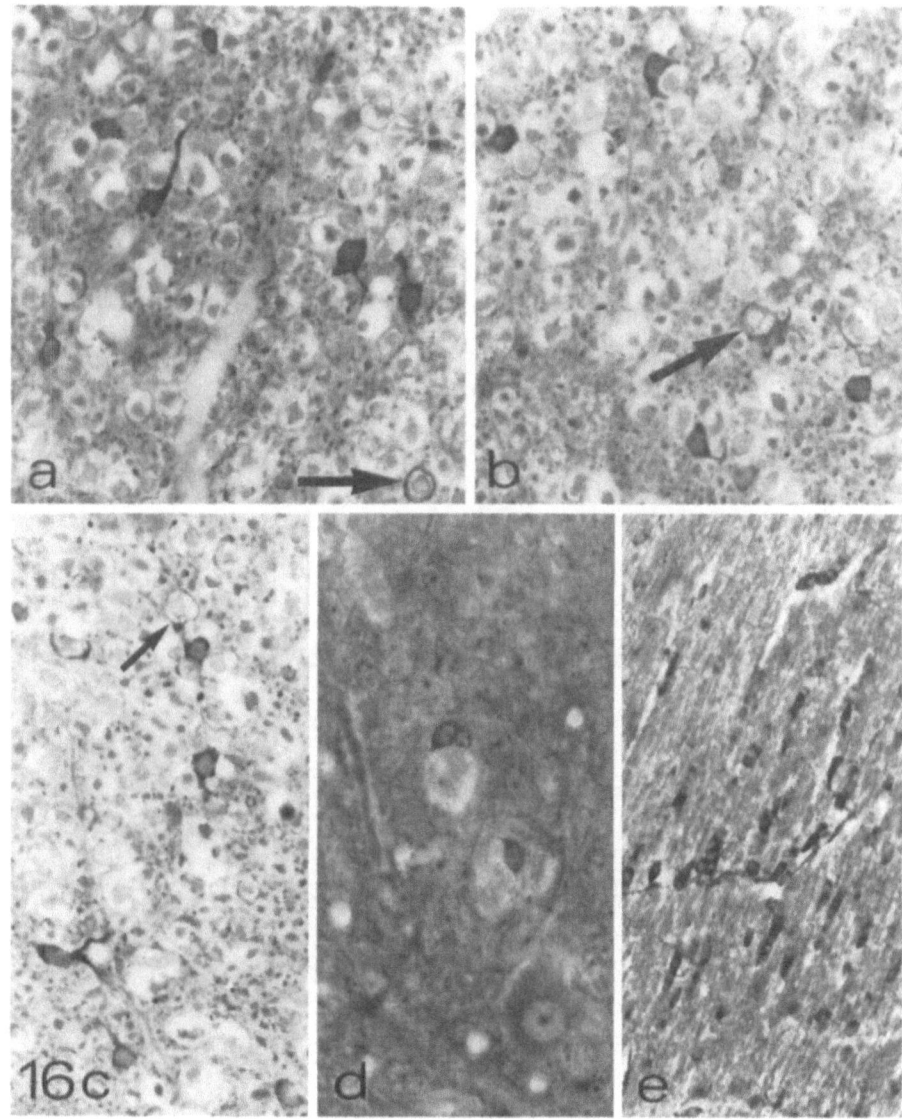

Fig. 16 a–e. Weil-Davenport impregnation technique for oligodendrocytes in normal white matter of EAE animals, showing specific impregnation of oligodendroglia cells and processes and impregnation of inner and outer oligendroglia loop of myelin sheaths *(arrows).* x 800. **a–c** Guinea pig spinal cord white matter. **d** Perineuronal satellite cells in guinea pig spinal cord gray matter. **e** Interfascicular oligendroglia in the centrum semiovale of the guinea pig

49

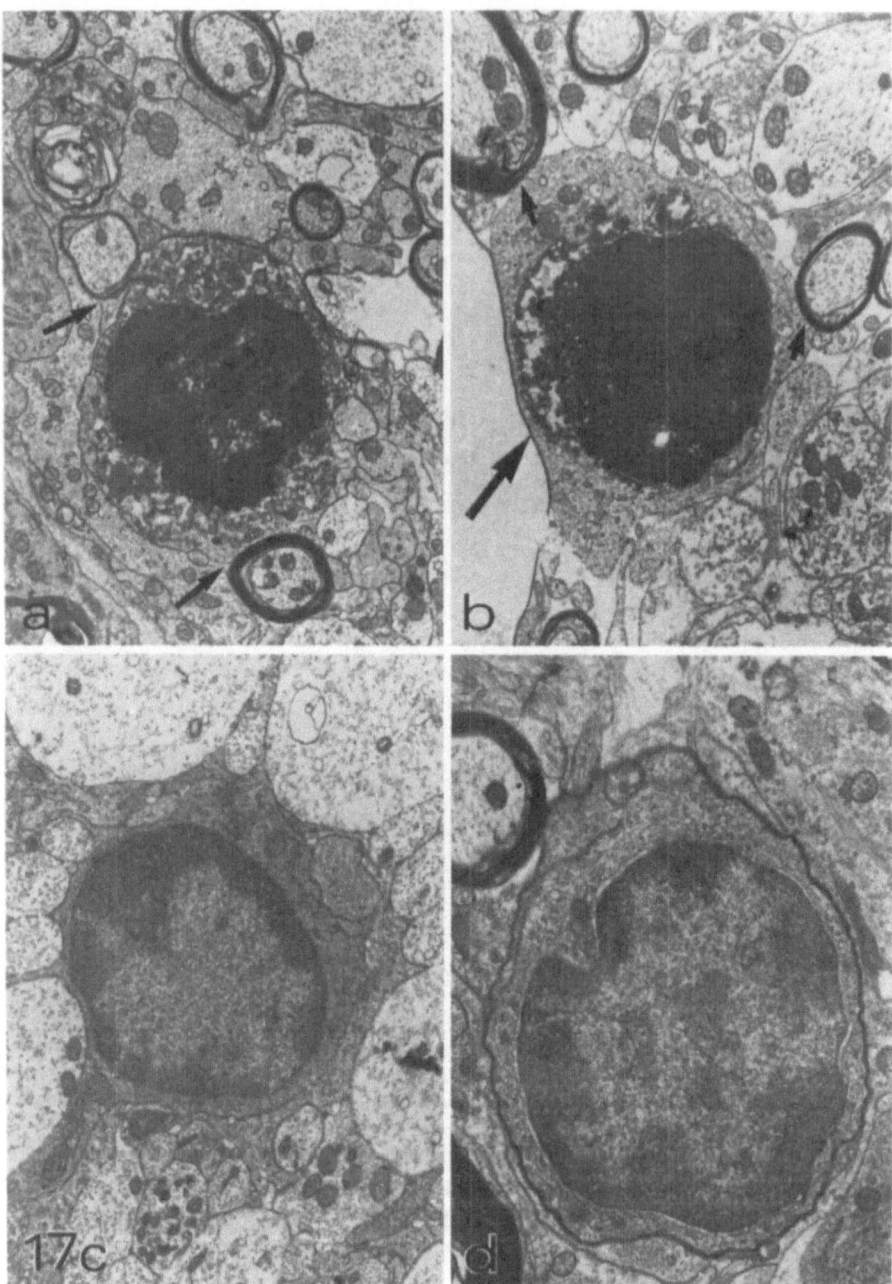

Fig. 17 a–d. Oligodendroglia in chronic EAE lesions in Hartley guinea pigs. **a** Border zone of an actively demyelinating lesion; degenerating cell, probably oligodendrocyte, still closely related to adjacent myelinated fibers *(arrows)*. EM, x 8300. **b** Border of an actively demyelinating EAE lesion; degenerating cell with close contacts to adjacent myelin sheaths *(small arrows)*. On the *left (large arrow)* the outer lamellae of a largely balloned myelin sheath are in close contact with the degenerating cell. EM, x 8300. **c** Apparently unaffected oligodendrocyte in in active demyelinated plaque. EM, x 8300. **d** Aberrant remyelination around an oligodendrocyte in a remyelinated plaque. EM x 9750

50

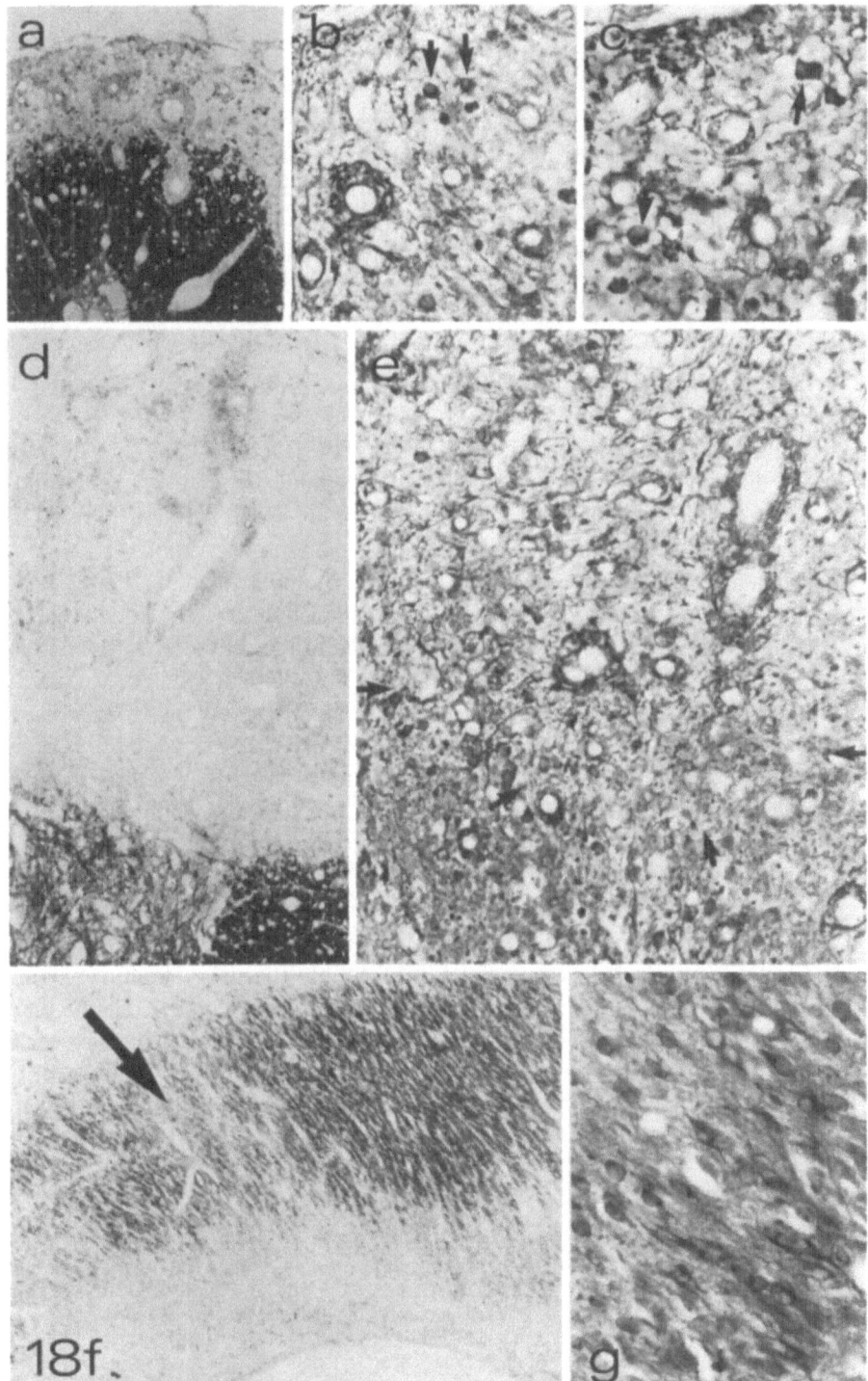

Fig. 18 a–g. Legend see page 52

51

All these observations suggest that in EAE myelin is the primary target in the pathogenesis of plaque formation. As myelin and oligodendrocytes share some antigens, these cells may be secondarily destroyed to a variable extent in an immunological attack directed against myelin. This view is further supported by the fact that sensitization with oligodendrocyte preparations results in a disease morphologically identical to that found after sensitization with white matter or myelin (Raine et al. 1977). Furthermore, the encephalogenic activity of oligodendrocyte fractions apparently depends upon the content of myelin basic protein in the preparation (McDermott et al. 1977).

4.5.2 Oligodendroglia in Multiple Sclerosis

In multiple sclerosis the exact determination of the fate of oligodendrocytes is even more difficult than with EAE, because in addition to the above-mentioned problems of identification the generally poor tissue preservation of autopsy material casts doubt on the significance of ultrastructural observations.

On a light microscopic level McAlpine (1955) and Lumsden (1970) described reduction or loss of oligodendroglia cells in MS plaques and concluded that these cells are destroyed simultaneously with myelin during active demyelination. This view was challenged by Ibrahim and Adams (1963, 1965) in detailed histochemical studies on oligodendroglia in MS comparing quantitatively histology with silver impregnation techniques and enzyme histochemistry. These studies revealed several interesting aspects: Oligodendrocytes were consistently reduced in number in several large plaques, but were increased in lesions with a diameter of less than $0.1\,mm^2$. The reduction of oligodendrocytes in large plaques was variable, ranging from less than 10% up to 80% compared with normal white matter. Furthermore, an up to twofold increase of oligodendrocytes was noted at the periphery of active as well as inactive plaques. Rows of interfascicular oligodendrocytes were noted at the plaque margins, extending some distance into the demyelinating lesions.

Whereas there is little controversy about the variable degree of oligodendroglia reduction in the center of large demyelinated plaques in MS, the increase of these cells at the plaque margin has been questioned in later investigations (Lumsden 1970). The higher amount of oxidative enzyme activity which can be consistently

---

◁ **Fig. 18 a–g.** Chronic lesions in the guinea pig, early chronic stage of the disease. **a** Actively demyelinating lesion with recent myelin degradation products. Klüver, x 50. **b, c** Same lesion as in **a**; Weil-Davenport silver impregnation for oligodendrocytes. Oligodendrocytes seem to be partly preserved in the lesions *(arrows)*. Some impregnation of debris-containing phagocytes, in addition. **b** x 690, **c** x 785. **d** Inactive early chronic lesion with initial remyelination. Klüver, x 80. **e** Same area impregnated for oligodendrocytes; some reduction of oligodendrocytes. The number of oligodendrocytes is reduced compared with the normal white matter in the lower portions *(border labeled by arrows)* of the micrograph. x 490. **f** Periventricular demyelinated plaque with large area of shadow plaque appearance *(arrow)*. Klüver, x 50. **g** Oligodendroglia impregnation in shadow plaque; a high number of impregnated interfascicular oligodendrocytes can be seen. x 980

noted at the plaque borders (Friede 1961; Ibrahim and Adams 1963, 1965; Lassmann 1969) may be explained by reactive changes in cells in actively demyelinating lesions or by remyelination, which, as will be discussed below, is frequently noted in these regions. Furthermore, as silver stains are only of limited specificity, some activated microglia cells may be misinterpreted as oligodendrocytes.

Ultrastructural investigations have contributed little to our knowledge about oligodendrocyte behavior in MS. At the borders of active and inactive lesions some increase of oligodendroglia size and some vacuolation of the cytoplasm has been noted (Field and Raine 1964; Perier and Gregoire 1965; Suzuki et al. 1969; Rinne et al. 1972). These changes are best interpreted as reactive alterations due to edema. Also the absence of oligodendrocytes from the center of old sclerotic lesions has been described (Sluga 1969). More recently Raine et al. (1981a, b) confirmed the relative preservation of interfascicular oligodendrocytes at the borders of active MS lesions.

In an immunohistochemical study of the distribution of myelin basic protein and myelin-associated glycoprotein in MS lesions, Itoyama et al. (1980) suggested that the formation of MS lesions is due to a primary defect of oligodendrocytes. This study, however, is based on a small number of cases and lesions. Furthermore, there is no definitive evidence available yet that reduction of myelin-associated glycoprotein in all instances reflects a dysfunction of oligodendrocytes.

Our own light and electron microscopic studies on acute and chronic MS may explain to some extent the divergent opinions about the fate of oligodendrocytes in this disease. Even when the same precautions regarding the identification of these cells, which have been discussed already in EAE, are considered, there seem to be differences in the extent of oligodendroglia destruction between small lesions of acute and rapidly progressive chronic MS compared with the typical large plaques of chronic MS. In a general pattern oligodendrocytes are most effectively destroyed in the large lesions of chronic MS although even in this situation a plaque completely free of oligodendroglia-like cells is rare. In acute and rapidly progressing chronic MS, cells resembling oligodendroglia may be present in inactive completely demyelinated plaques in numbers, comparable to those in normal periplaque white matter. Furthermore, as will be discussed below, remyelination seems to be pronounced in acute MS lesions occurring within a few days to weeks after formation of the plaque.

In summary, the fate of oligodendroglia in MS and EAE lesions will not be elucidated without reservations until detailed studies with specific oligodendroglia markers are available. However, our present light and electron microscopic evidence indicates that there is no cytopathic change of oligodendrocytes which precedes demyelination. Thus, both diseases do not seem to be primary disorders of oligodendrocytes. This is further supported by the patterns of demyelination with myelin stripping and vesicular disruption of myelin, suggesting that myelin is the main target in the pathogenesis of the disease. Oligodendrocytes as a functional unit with myelin sheath may degenerate to a variable extent during active deymelination.

4.6 Remyelination

The importance of remyelination as a repair mechanism in the central nervous system has been recognized during the past 20 years with the use of the electron microscope in human and experimental neuropathology. Extensive or even complete remyelination is now well documented, occurring in many experimental models (Bunge et al. 1961; Lampert 1965, 1967; Hirano et al. 1968; Prineas et al. 1969; Wisniewski and Raine 1971; Blakemore 1973, 1975; Ludwin 1978, 1980). In human neuropathology, especially in multiple sclerosis, remyelination may be present (Feigin and Popoff 1966; Suzuki et al. 1969; Ogata and Feigin 1975; Prineas and Connel 1979). It is, however, still considered by many authors as a rare phenomenon which does not contribute significantly to functional repair of demyelinated lesions (Lumsden 1970). This view seems to be partly due to difficulties in the identification of remyelination in tissue obtained from autopsy, performed several hours after death. Furthermore, little is known about the time course of remyelination in human demyelinating diseases. Thus the study of the dynamics of remyelination in chronic relapsing EAE may help us to understand the factors regulating the extent of remyelination, not only in the experimental model but also in the human disease.

4.6.1 Remyelination in Acute and Chronic EAE

The presence of remyelination in EAE has been well established since the earliest descriptions by Lapert (1965, 1967). Furthermore, in the demyelinated lesions in chronic models of EAE the repair of myelin by oligodendrocytes and Schwann cells (Snyder et al. 1975a) frequently leads to nearly complete remyelination in the lesions (Raine et al. 1978a; Lassmann and Wisniewski 1979a). A more detailed study of lesional morphology in chronic relapsing EAE in Hartley guinea pigs, however, reveals at first view a paradoxical situation. Remyelination is much more pronounced in animals sampled during the early chronic stage of the disease (40–100 dps) than in those investigated in the late chronic stage (100–200 dps). Only in later stages after sensitization (300 dps and later) is remyelination again the dominating feature of lesional pathology. This unexpected finding seems to be due to differences in the extent and velocity of remyelination in different stages of the disease, depending mainly on the time interval between sensitization and plaque formation (Lassmann et al. 1980b). In lesions formed during the subacute and early chronic stage of the disease (20–100 dps), remyelination by oligodendrocytes is very rapid and extensive (Fig. 19). According to clinicopathological correlation in these stages of the disease initial remyelination may be noted as early as 6 days after plaque formation. In these lesions and those investigated during the following

2 weeks many axons in the plaques are surrounded by thin myelin sheaths of uniform thickness. In electron microscopy all stages of active remyelination with noncompacted myelin sheaths and irregularities in the ensheathment can be found (Fig. 20). Intermingled between these remyelinating nerve fibers numerous phagocytes, containing all (even the earliest) stages of myelin debris, are still found. When the debris-containing phagocytes are removed, these lesions either have the appearance of hypomyelination, similar to shadow plaques in MS, or when studied at later time intervals, may even be completely remyelinated. In the latter situation the extension of the previously demyelinated plaque can be identified only by the presence of gliosis and perivenous and pericapillary fibrosis. Schwann cell remyelination is extremely rare in early chronic lesions.

A different picture is encountered when plaques are studied which were formed during the late chronic stage of the disease (100–200 dps) (Fig, 21). In these lesions central (oligodendroglial) remyelination is sparse, mainly located at the lesional borders, and only found late after plaque formation, with an interval of demyelination and remyelination of up to several months. Thus in general in these lesions the simultaneous presence of phagocytes with myelin degradation products and remyelinated nerve fibers was not observed, and the classical lesion in this stage is the demyelinated sclerotic plaque. Furthermore, invasion of Schwann cells into demyelinated plaques of the spinal cord and partial peripheral remyelination is a common observation in lesions formed during the late chronic stage of the disease (Fig. 21).

The time course of remyelination during the early chronic stage of chronic relapsing EAE follows closely that found in other experimental models of demylination (Gledhill et al. 1973; Gledhill and Mc Donald 1977; Herndon et al. 1975; Ludwin 1978) and in acute EAE (Lampert 1965). This observation is different from others previously described in EAE, where the onset of remyelination was found much later after lesion formation (Prineas et al. 1969), similar to that in the late chronic stage of chronic relapsing EAE. According to our observations in chronic relapsing EAE, the velocity and extent of remyelination decrease with the time interval between sensitization and plaque formation.

There are several possible explanations for this phenomenon. As has been discussed above the extent of oligodendroglia destruction also increases with the time

---

Fig. 19 a–e. Remyelination in the early chronic phase of chronic relapsing EAE. **a.** Large, sharply demar- ▷ cated plaque in the dorsal regions of the cord; recent active lesion, subpial in the anterior and lateral columns. Klüver, x 30. **b** Higher magnification of lesion in the anterior columns; numerous droplets of myelin degradation products in the lesion. Klüver, x 250. **c** Lesion in the dorsal column with faintly stained thin myelin sheaths. Klüver, x 250. **d, e** Early active lesion in the spinal cord of an animal from the early chronic phase of the disease (45 dps); presence of earliest stages of myelin degradation in the lesion *(arrows);* the nerve fibers in the lesions contain thin myelin sheaths of uniform thickness indicating rapid remyelination. **d** Toluidine blue, x 300; **e** Toluidine blue, x 1000

Fig. 20. Electron micrograph of a remyelinating early chronic lesion; partly uncompacted myelin. EM, x ▷▷ 15000

55

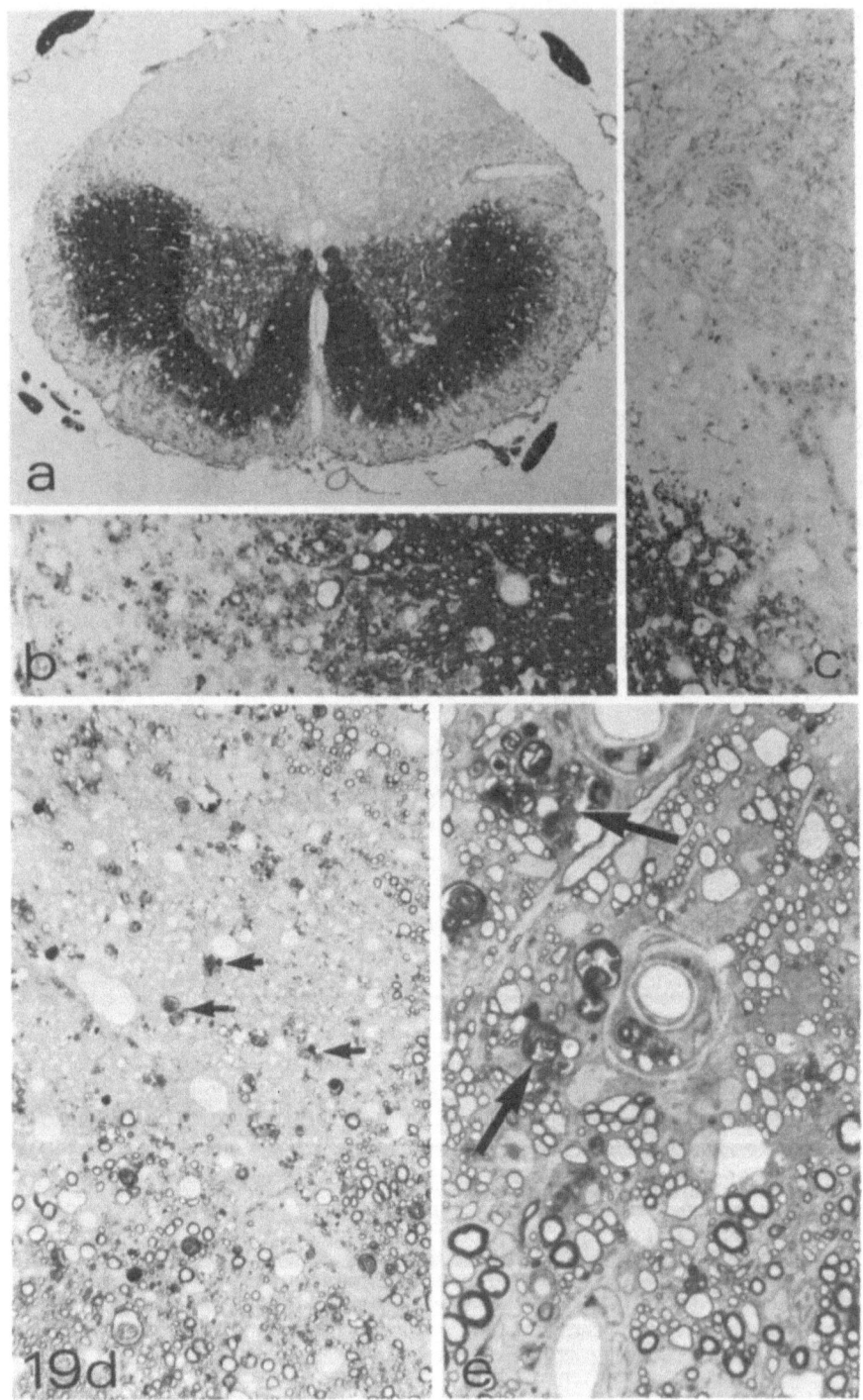

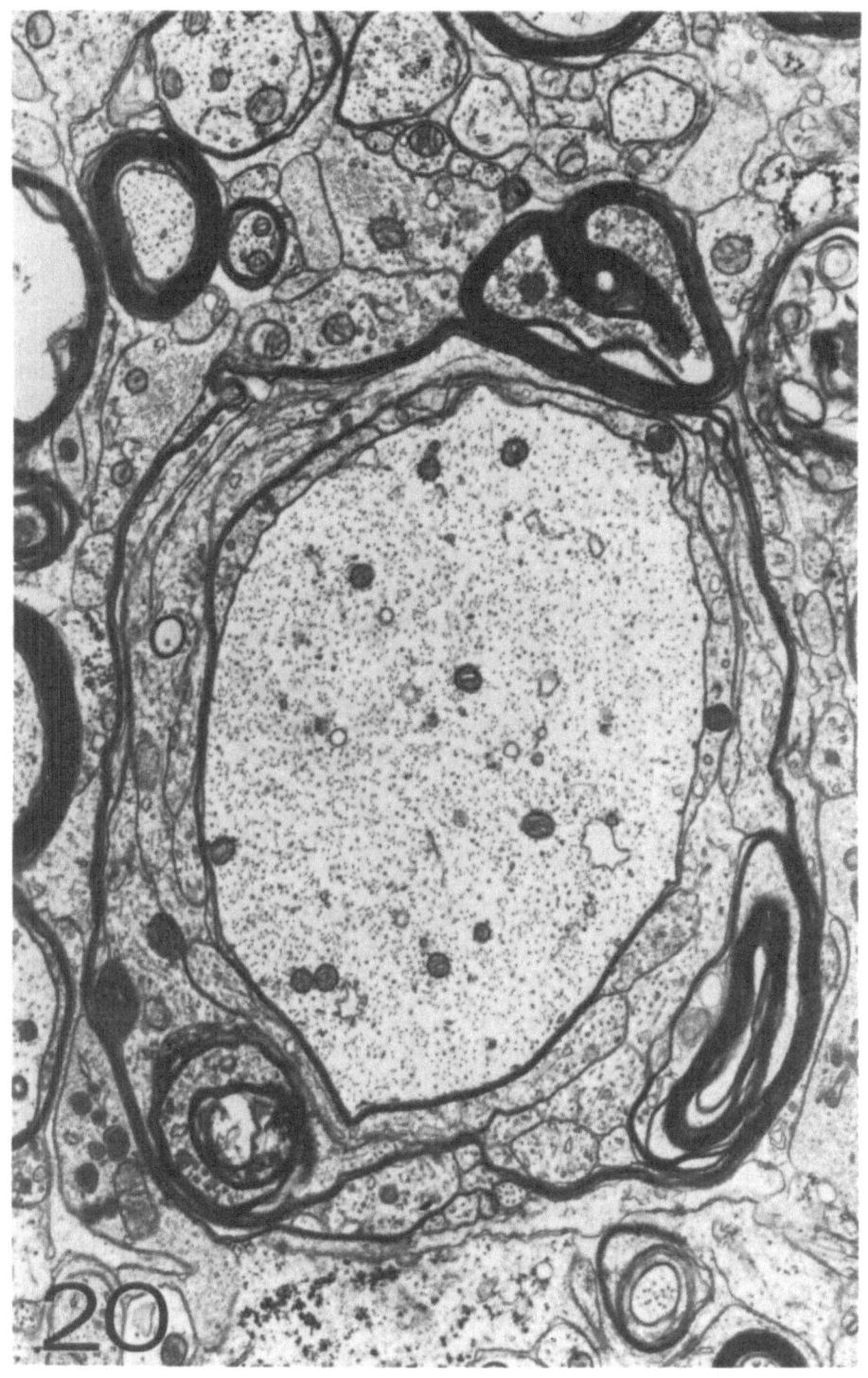

interval between sensitization and plaque formation. Thus in late chronic lesions less oligodendrocytes are available for remyelination in the lesions than in early chronic plaques. The availability of oligodendrocytes seems to be one of the most important limiting factors regulating the degree of remyelination, at least in cuprizone-induced demyelinated lesions (Ludwin 1980). Also gliosis is more pronounced in late chronic, compared with early chronic lesions. Some evidence from in vitro studies suggests that gliosis may also have an inhibiting effect on remyelination in vitro (Raine and Bornstein 1970b) although in vivo the degree of gliosis did not influence the extent of remyelination (Ludwin 1980). Furthermore, antibodies directed against myelin components may inhibit remyelination, as suggested from in vitro studies (Bornstein and Raine 1970; Seil et al. 1973, 1975). Thus it is interesting that in chronic relapsing EAE intrathecally synthesized immunoglobulins increase with time after sensitization, reaching maximal levels between 100 and 200 dps (Mehta et al. 1980, 1981). It is at present unresolved whether these antibodies are directed against myelin or oligodendroglia antigens.

Remyelination by Schwann cells is mainly a feature of late chronic lesions, and is only infrequently found in animals sampled up to the 100th day after sensitization (Fig. 21). According to other models of demyelination in the spinal cord (as e.g., demyelination following lysolecithin injections into the cerebrospinal fluid or following-X-irradiation), the extent of peripheral remyelination is dependent upon the degree of damage to astrocytes, especially in the region of the glia limitans (Blakemore 1975, 1976; Blakemore and Paterson 1975). Similar irregularities in the glia limitans can also be found in late chronic EAE lesions (Raine et al. 1978b; Lassmann et al. 1981b) (Fig. 21). Furthermore, the most vigorous peripheral remyelination was found in rare destructive demyelinated plaques in the spinal cord of rats suffering from chronic EAE, in lesions where astrocytes were nearly completely damaged and destroyed during the formation of the plaques (Lassmann et al. 1980b).

Simultaneous presence of active demyelination and active remyelination is a rare phenomenon in EAE lesions. In demyelinated plaques, especially in the early chronic stage of the disease (40–100 dps), active plaque growth at one edge may sometimes be combined with remyelination in other areas. In these lesions, however, actively demyelinating and remyelinating areas are separated by a demyelinated inactive zone. Moreover, in such lesions it cannot be excluded that active demyelination involves a previously de- and remyelinated area. In rare instances, active demyelination of central (oligodendroglial) myelin in late chronic lesions may be found in the immediate vicinity of peripheral (Schwann cell) remyelination. In these cases the immunological reaction seems to be restricted to central myelin without affecting myelin produced by Schwann cells.

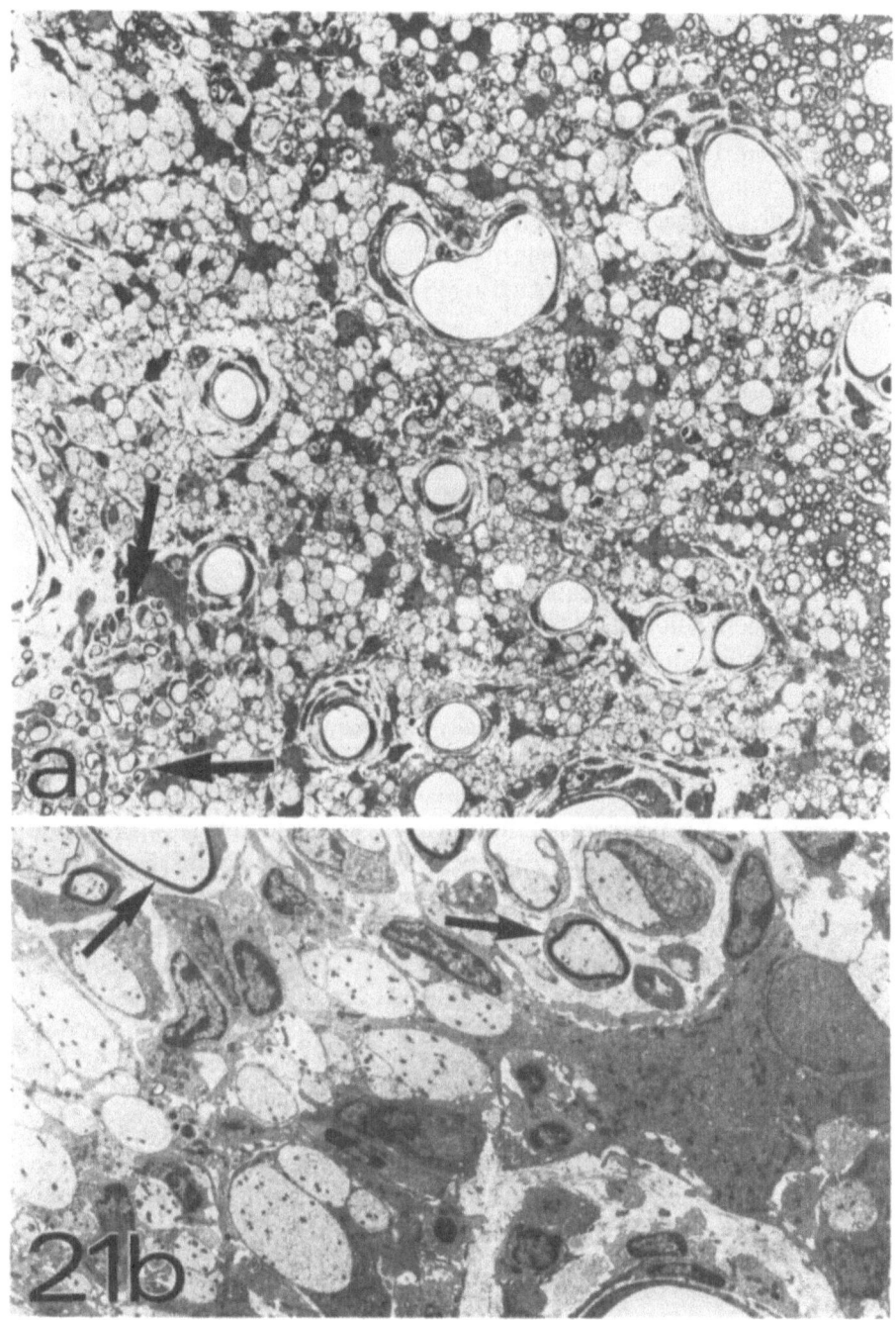

Fig. 21 a, b. Demyelinated plaque in the late chronic stage of chronic relapsing EAE. **a** Extensive gliosis and lack of remyelination; in a small area peripheral remyelination can be seen in a region where the glia limiting membrane is defective *(arrows)*. EM, ×490. **b** Higher magnification of **a**; peripheral remyelination *(arrows)* together with marked reactive gliosis and defective glia limitans. EM, ×2425

4.6.2 Remyelination in Multiple Sclerosis

The occurrence of remyelination in multiple sclerosis plaques has been described by several authors. Remyelination may be performed by oligodendrocytes (Perier and Gregoire 1965; Suzuki et al. 1969; Prineas and Connel 1979) as well as by Schwann cells (Feigin and Popoff 1966; Andrews 1972; Ghatak et al. 1973). In these studies remyelination has been documented at the margins of chronic inactive lesions in MS. A functionally more significant question, however, is whether whole plaques may be remyelinated in MS and at what time interval remyelination may follow plaque formation.

The occurrence of shadow plaques is a characteristic finding in MS pathology (Lumsden 1970). There are several possible explanations for the development of shadow plaques in MS.

Areas of white matter pallor may be found in acute and chronic edema of the white matter. In MS, however, edematous changes in the chronic stage are generally not pronounced and severe edema may only be present in actively demyelinating lesions.

Another possible explanation for reduction of myelinated fibers is partial axonal destruction in fiber tracts in the CNS. This may occur frequently in MS, especially in long tracts in the spinal cord and brain stem. Both mechanisms, edema and incomplete tract degeneration, do not explain the presence of irregularly shaped sclerotic shadow plaques topographically oriented to veins of the CNS, which are especially frequent in MS pathology.

Lumsden (1970) introduced the concept of incomplete demyelination in active MS plaques as an explanation for the appearance of shadow plaques. This interpretation is based mainly upon two observations: The abundance of shadow plaques in acute MS, even in cases with a clinical history of a few weeks only, and the presence of the earliest stages of myelin debris in some of the shadow lesions. Both findings, however, may be alternatively interpreted as rapid remyelination similar to our observation in the early chronic stage of chronic relapsing EAE.

The fourth possible mechanism for the formation of shadow plaques is remyelination of previously demyelinated lesions. As will be discussed below, our results indicate that the majority of these lesions are due to remyelination.

The incidence of shadow plaques in MS brains varies from case to case. In acute MS (Marburg's type) shadow lesions are especially frequent. In some cases even no lesions can be found where myelin is completely absent. In chronic MS cases the typical lesion is the sharply demarcated sclerotic demyelinated plaque. Shadow plaques, although present in variable numbers, are rare compared with acute MS.

Myelin degradation products in shadow plaques — sometimes even in the earliest stages — are frequently present in acute MS. In chronic MS, however, in our material active lesions with initial stages of myelin degradation products did not contain myelinated fibers. The sequence of events leading to the formation of shadow plaques can best be studied in cases of chronic MS with short duration of the disease (2–3 years) (Fig. 22). In lesions of these patients, small clusters of thinly myelinated nerve fibers first appear during the sudanophilic stage of myelin degradation simultaneously with the onset of fibrillary sclerosis. In the same brain, later lesions, which still contain a few PAS-positive degradation products and already show marked fibrillary sclerosis, appear as areas of myelin pallor with uniform distribution of thinly myelinated fibers throughout the whole plaque area. Shadow plaques, which do not contain myelin degradation products, are characterized by a decreased density of myelinated fibers, indicating some axonal loss, and by myelin sheaths which are still thinner than those in the surrounding white matter. In addition to these lesions there are several patchy areas of fibrillary sclerosis and vascular fibrosis with apparently normal myelin density and myelin sheath thickness. According to their shape and distribution these lesions are comparable to other demyelinated or shadow plaques and thus may represent areas of complete remyelination.

As mentioned above thin myelin sheaths within the whole plaque may be found simultaneously with the presence of earliest stages of myelin debris in acute MS. In these lesions thus a discrimination between incomplete demyelination and remyelination is more difficult. Myelin sheaths in these plaques are very thin, with uniform myelin thickness, and are frequently arranged in clusters apparently following the distribution of preserved oligodendrocytes. In acute MS lesions which contain later stages of myelin debris (sudanophilic or PAS-positive), a gradient of myelin sheath thickness can be found with extremely thin sheaths in the center, the thickness of myelin increasing toward the periphery of the lesion. In later stages of plaque development when myelin debris is removed, a similar appearance of shadow plaques is noted in acute MS, as described before in chronic MS.

Electron microscopy of shadow plaques in acute as well as chronic MS confirms the presence of nerve fibers with disproportionately thin myelin sheaths. Furthermore, some irregularities in the ensheathment of axons can be seen, with the appearance of uncompacted myelin and aberrant myelin loops.

In summary, the above-described observations indicate the following implications for the interpretation of MS lesions:

1. Remyelination may take place in multiple sclerosis not only in a limited zone of the plaque border but may even represent a repair mechanism for whole plaques.

2. The extent of remyelination in MS varies from case to case. As a general rule, however, lesions from cases with short clinical history, especially acute MS cases, tend to remyelinate more effectively than those from chronic cases.

3. Remyelination may start rapidly after plaque formation, especially in cases of acute MS. This may lead to the simultaneous presence of the earliest myelin degradation products together with remyelination in the same lesions. With chronicity of the disease, not only the extent but also the velocity of remyelination decreases in newly formed lesions.

4. Although definite proof is still lacking, our results indicate that complete re-myelination may occur in MS, resulting in patchy areas of fibrillary gliosis and vascular fibrosis with no apparent difference in myelin density. This may also explain the frequent observation of gliosis in the otherwise apparently normal white matter in this disease (Allen and McKeown 1979; Allen et al. 1981).

5. Rapid and extensive remyelination in acute and early chronic MS may partly explain the rapid and complete clinical recovery of patients after the first exacerbations of the disease. Remyelination, however, does not necessarily result in a measurable improvement of function, because axonal loss may be pronounced in shadow plaques.

4.7 Sclerosis

As expressed in the name of the disease, the formation of a dense glial scar in multiple sclerosis is one of the most characteristic aspects of lesional structure. Gliosis, however, is not a feature unique for MS plaques but a common repair mechanism following CNS injury. Furthermore, demyelinating diseases with pathogenesis distinctly different from that of MS may show similar dense glial scar formation. There are, however, several aspects of gliosis in MS which have attracted attention since the earliest descriptions of the disease by Charcot (1868). Gliosis occurs very early during plaque formation (Charcot 1868; Müller 1904; Hallervorden 1940; Lumsden 1970). In inactive plaques the increase of astrocytes and their fibrillary processes is frequently not restricted to the plaque area itself but may extend a considerable distance into the surrounding apparently normal white matter. These astrocytes in the plaque and periplaque areas contain an increased amount of proteolytic enzymes which are considered to act as mediators in the demyelinating process (Mc Keown and Allen 1979). It has therefore still not been settled whether gliosis in MS is a primary event in the disease, contributing to the pathogenesis of demyelination, or whether it merely represents a consequence of tissue destruction. As in the late phase of chronic relapsing EAE gliosis similar to that found in MS (Lassmann and Wisniewski 1979a) is present, the dynamics of glial scar formation in this model may help to interpret the above-mentioned questions.

Fig. 22 a–f. Remyelination in multiple sclerosis. 34–year-old-female with chronic relapsing MS, leading ▷ to death 4 years after onset of the disease. Multiple small- to medium-sized partly active, partly inactive, or shadow plaques throughout the whole brain in autospy; plaques of different ages in the frontal white matter. **a, b** Active lesion with earliest myelin degradation products; note the complete absence of myelinated fibers in the lesion. **a** Klüver, x 300; **b** Toluidine, x 500. **c, d** Plaque in the sudanophilic stage of myelin degradation; shadow appearance of the lesion with occurrence of numerous thin myelin sheaths **c** or appearance of small clusters of thinly myelinated fibers in the center of the lesion **d**; macrophages with myelin degradating products are labeled with *arrows*. **c** Klüver-PAS, x 300; **d** Toluidine blue, x 1000. **e, f** Shadow plaques with reactive gliosis and absence of myelin degradation products. **e** Klüver-PAS, x 300; **f** Toluidine blue, x 500

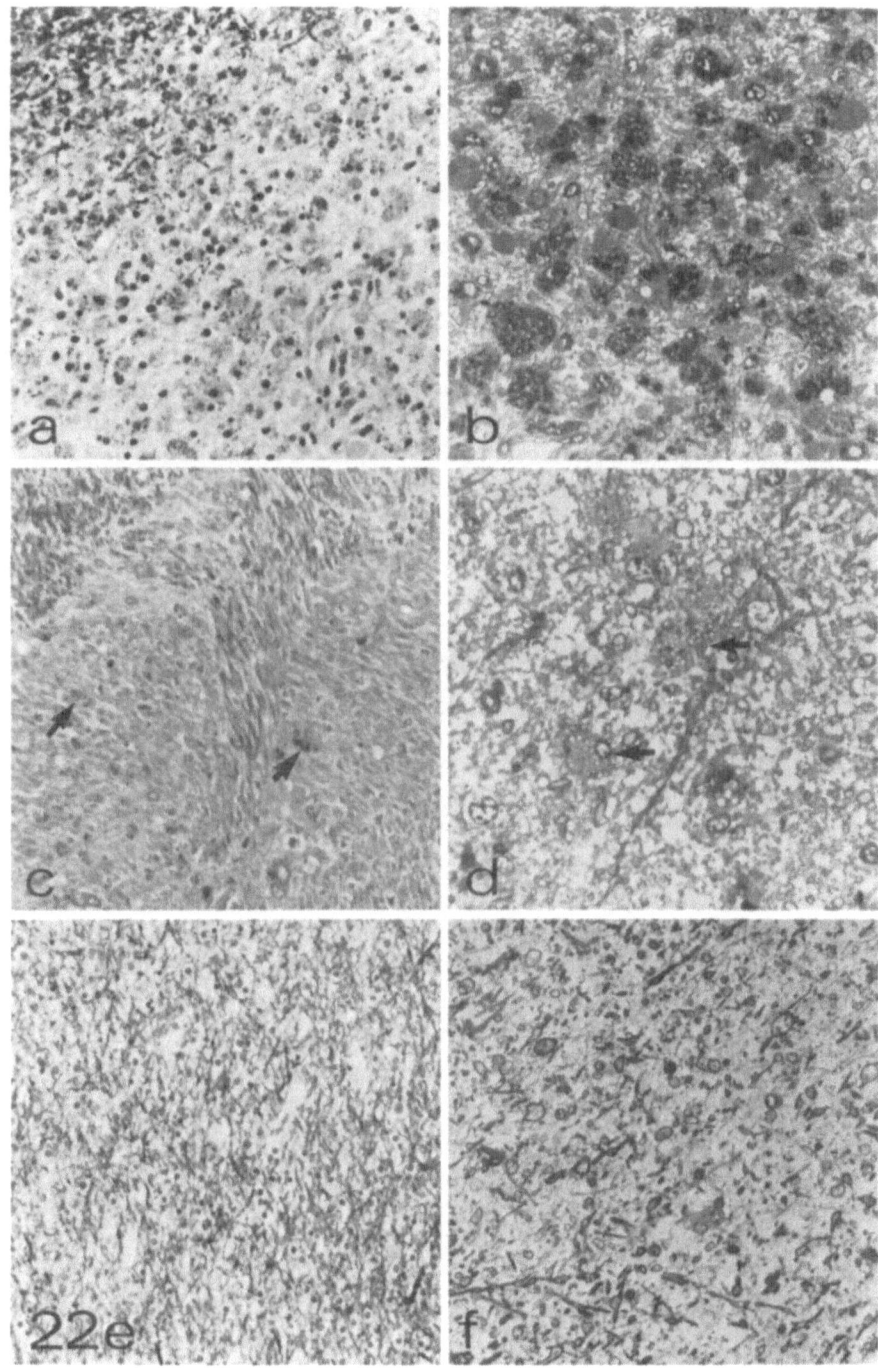

63

4.7.1 Astroglial Reaction in the Lesions of Acute and Chronic EAE

In experimental allergic encephalomyelitis the astroglial reaction was believed for a long time to be different from that found in multiple sclerosis. Acute EAE lesions, even when studied a long time after the active stage of the disease, did not show comparable fibrillary gliosis at the light and electron microscopic level (Morgan 1946; Wolf et al. 1947). In a more chronic model of EAE in monkeys, Ferraro and Cazzullo (1948) described an increase of astroglial cells and some patchy fibrillar gliosis. The glia reaction, however, was not confined to the demyelinated lesions and was most pronounced in old necrotic foci in the gray and white matter. In contrast in chronic EAE some increase of astrocytes was shown with the electron microscope by Raine et al. (1974), and dense, light microscopically visible, fibrillar glial scars were regularly found in late stages after sensitization (Lassmann and Wisniewski 1979a). When gliosis in chronic relapsing EAE is studied, it is important to differentiate between lesions formed at different time intervals after sensitization.

In lesions formed in the acute or subacute stage of the disease (10–40 days after sensitization), the leading pathological picture is perivenous inflammation. Some perivenous demyelination is found in lesions which are formed or still active between the 20th and 30th day after sensitization. In these perivenous demyelinated areas, even when studied several weeks after their formation, in animals with a very long remission after the acute or subacute disease episode, gliosis is absent or mild. Ultrastructurally some increase in perivascular astrocytes may be found together with thickened cellular processes which contain bundles of glial fibrils.

Lesions which are formed during the early chronic phase of the disease (40–100 days after sensitization) are characterized by intense perivenous inflammation, plaque-like demyelination with relative preservation of oligodendrocytes and rapid remyelination. In these plaques, similar to in those in acute and subacute lesions, gliosis is absent during the active stage of demyelination, which is characterized by the presence of myelin debris. Astroglial scar formation may be found 14–30 days at the earliest after plaque formation and is relatively mild. It consists of an increase of astrocytic nuclei together with the formation of a loose network of cellular processes which separate individual nerve fiber bundles. At the light microscopic level this fibrillar network is best visualized in PTAH-stained sections, however, in Holzers glia stain, affected areas are only moderately denser compared with the surrounding tissue. When such lesions are studied at later time intervals, at a stage when they are completely remyelinated, no further increase in the intensity of gliosis is found.

Late chronic lesions developing 100–200 days after sensitization can be best studied in animals with a long clinically silent period between the acute episode and the first relapse of the disease (Fig. 23). These lesions are characterized by a weaker inflammatory response than with early chronic plaques, by extensive plaquelike demyelination with considerable loss of oligodendrocytes and by only a

64

minor degree of central remyelination, which is generally confined to the lesional borders. Gliosis in these plaques is intense and can be found as early as 5–10 days after plaque formation at a stage where most recent myelin degradation products are still present. This astroglial scar is best visualized in paraffin sections stained with the Holzers glia stain (Fig. 23). It extends beyond the borders of the demyelinated areas, also affecting a zone of apparently unaffected white matter. When such lesions are studied sequentially, the first change in astroglia is the appearance of large, often multinucleated bizarre-shaped cells (Figs. 23c, 24). These cells are most numerous in lesions which still contain remnants of myelin debris. With further clearing of the plaques, cellular increase of astrocytes continues; however, the individual cells generally become smaller with a stellate or spindle-shaped appearance and with cell processes packed with glial fibrils (Fig. 23d–f).

However, studying different demyelinated plaques even within one animal, a striking difference in the extent and structural expression of gliosis may be noted. In general the most pronounced gliosis may be found in periventricular lesions and optic nerve plaques. Gliosis in demyelinated plaques in the spinal cord is comparatively less pronounced. In cortical plaques and in other lesions in the gray matter the astroglia reaction is mild and frequently not detectable at a light microscopic level.

Activation of astrocytes in the periplaque, well-myelinated white matter is a feature of lesions in animals sampled during the late chronic stage of the disease (later than 100 days sensitization). It may consist of an inrease in number and volume of astrocytes together with mitoses of these cells in the periphery of actively demyelinating lesions. This observation indicates that stimulation of astroglia may exceed the actual demyelinating plaque. The other type of gliosis in well-myelinated white matter is found in chronic inactive lesions, with fibrillary gliosis in areas in the vicinity of a demyelinating plaque. In these lesions, however, frequently marked vascular changes involving small veins as well as capillaries can be found, indicating that these areas are old repaired (remyelinated) lesions. It must be noted, however, that gliosis is not a general feature of the white matter in chronic EAE animals and that in the animals gliosis was never found preceding demyelination.

Fig. 23 a–f. Gliosis in chronic relapsing EAE. **a, b** Spinal cord lesion in an animal sampled in the late ▷ chronic stage of chronic relapsing EAE; extensive fibrillar gliosis in the demyelinated areas. **a** Klüver,x 10; **b** Holzer's glia stain, x 10. **c** Extensive gliosis with large protoplasmatic astrocytes in a recent periventricular demyelinated plaque. Toluidine blue, x 500. **d** Fibrillary gliosis in a recent spinal cord lesion. Holzer, x 250. **e** Intense fibrillary gliosis in an old periventricular lesion. PATH, x 250. **f** Adjacent periventricular normal white matter. PATH, x 250

Fig. 24. Gliosis in chronic relapsing EAE lesion in animal sampled during the late chronic stage of the ▷▷ disease; pronounced protoplasmatic gliosis and defects in the glia limitans. EM, x 1780

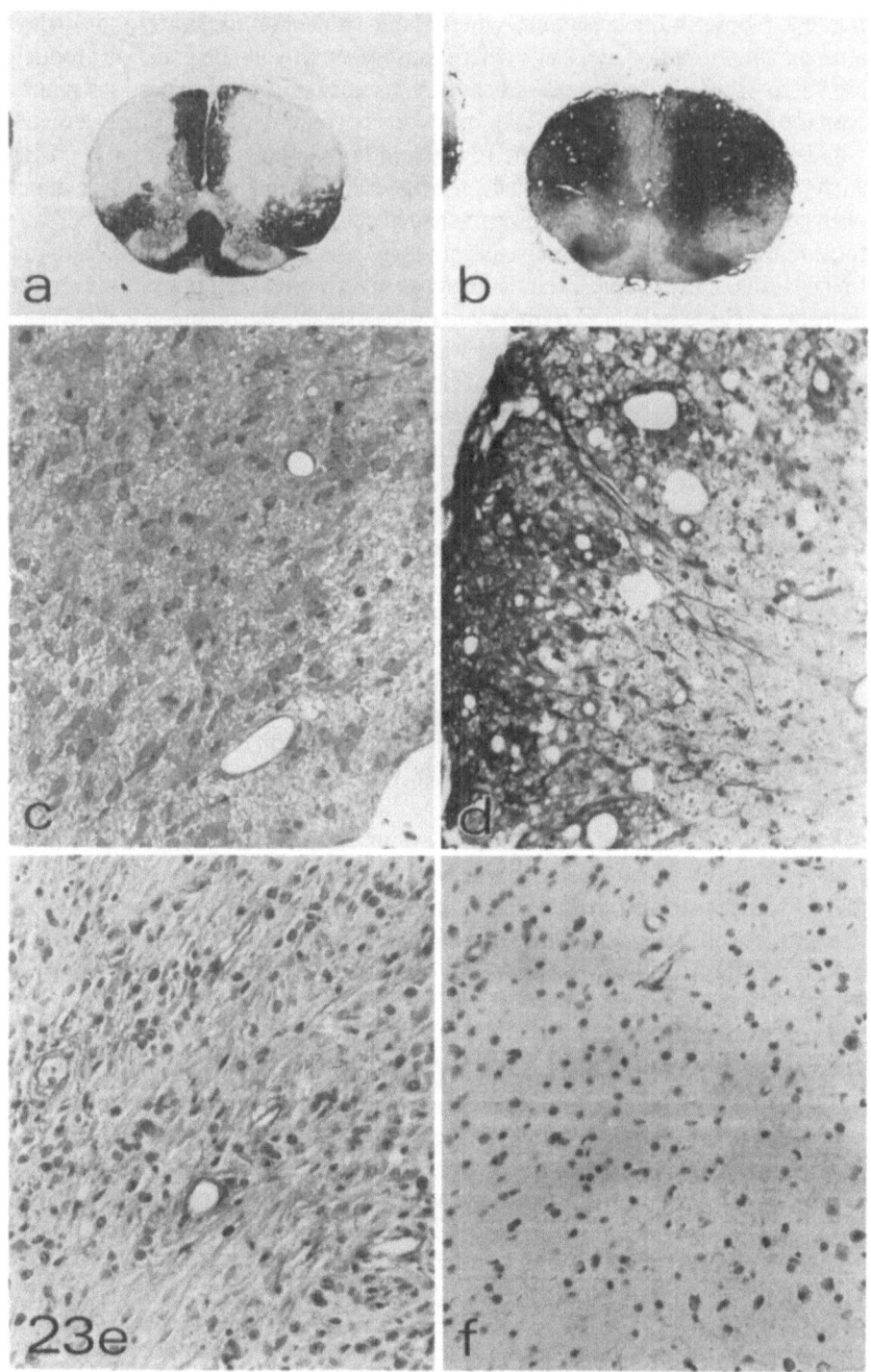

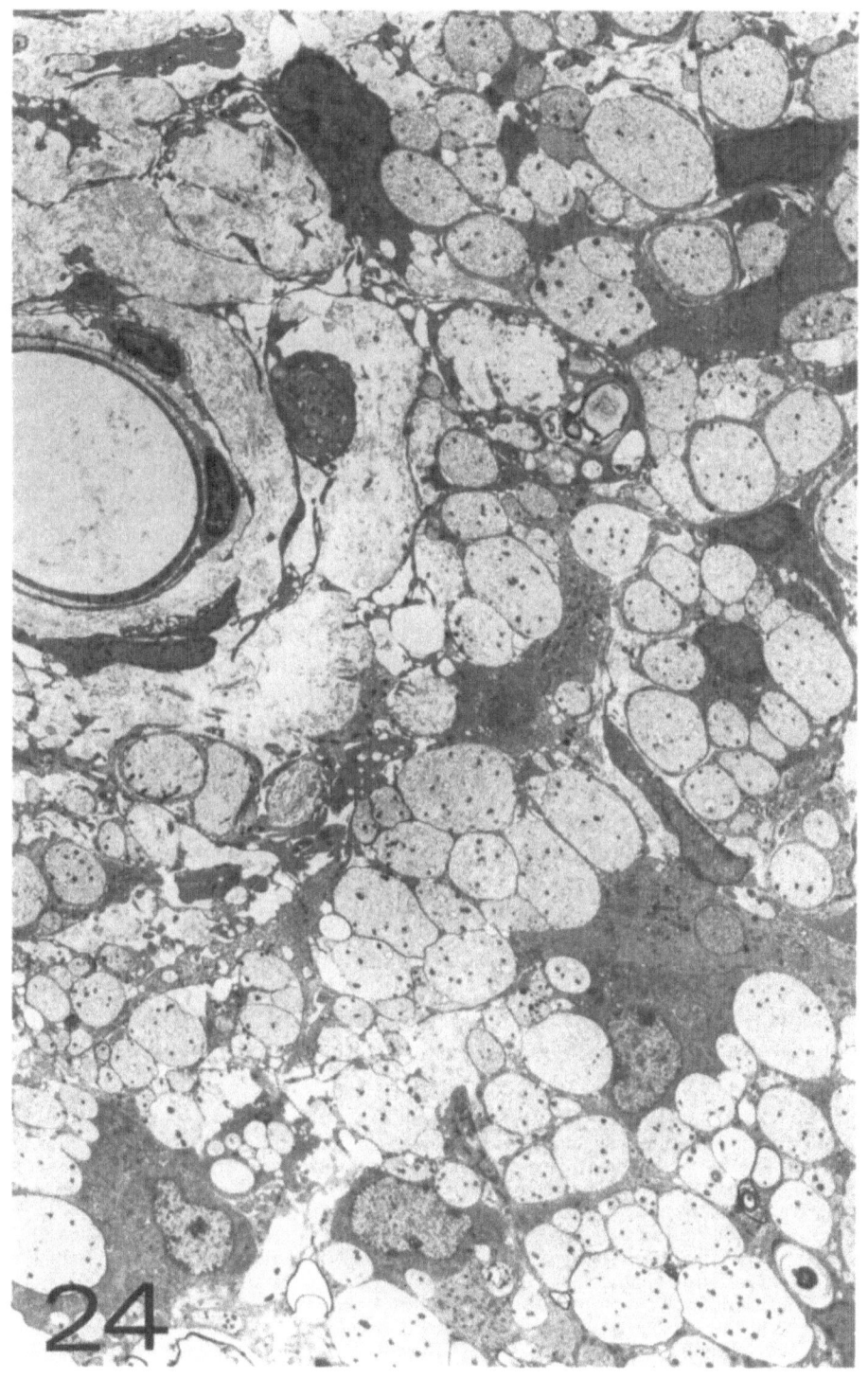

24

4.7.2 Gliosis in Multiple Sclerosis

It has been well known for decades that dense fibrillar gliosis within demyelinated plaques in multiple sclerosis is one of the most characteristic features of the lesions. There is, however, conflicting evidence regarding the time course and dynamics of glial scar formation. Studies which were mainly concerned with acute MS (Marburg 1906; Pette 1928; Siemerling and Raeke 1914; Adams 1977) revealed that in these cases gliosis is clearly a secondary event following demyelination (Fig. 25). Pette (1928) in his comparison of acute MS cases with different clinical durations found that light microscopically detectable gliosis was not found earlier than 14 days after plaque formation. Gliosis was first initiated by intense proliferation and increase in size of astrocytes leading to lesions packed with large bizarre, frequently multinucleated astrocytes (G. Peters 1935; Field et al. 1962) (Fig. 25), sometimes resembling the pathohistological picture of an astrocytoma (Rossolimo 1904; Strähuber 1903). This finding, however, does not imply a higher risk of neoplastic transformation of astrocytes in MS patients than in an age-matched control group (Lumsden 1970). At later stages after plaque formation a typical glial scar develops, consisting of smaller stellate- or spindle-shaped cells with processes packed with glial fibrils.

On the contrary, when active or inactive cases of typical chronic MS were studied, a different pattern of astroglial activation was found (Charcot 1868; Müller 1904; Anton and Wohlwill 1912; Hallervorden 1940; Field 1967) (Fig. 26). In active lesions in these cases gliosis was found to be a very early feature in plaque formation and was, frequently found simultaneously with active demyelination (Fig. 26) and even extending into the periplaque white matter. A similar glia activation in the well-myelinated white matter has also been found extending a considerable distance from the borders of chronic inactive MS lesions (Allen et al. 1979). No systematic studies regarding the influence of lesional topography in MS on the extent of sclerosis are available. It is, however, well established that in cortical plaques in MS gliosis is minimal or absent (Siemerling and Raeke 1914; Hallervorden 1940).

More recently it has been shown in immunohistochemical studies that many astrocytes in demyelinated plaques and also in the apparently normal white matter

---

Fig. 25 a–f. Gliosis in acute multiple sclerosis. **a, b** 26-year-old female with acute MS, leading to death 12 ▷ weeks after onset of the disease. **c–f** 30-year-old male, died from bronchopneumonia 2 weeks after onset of neurological disease; multiple small partly active demyelinated plaques in the internal capsule and brain stem. **a** Initial lesion with massive active demyelination absence of gliosis. Toluidine blue, x 1000. **b** Demyelinated lesion with ongoing activity; single large protoplasmatic astrocytes. Toluidine blue, x 1000. **c** Lesion in the sudanophilic stage of myelin degradation with the beginning of remyelination and massive protoplasmatic gliosis. Toluidine blue, x 1000. **d** Lesion in the sudanophilic and PAS-positive stage of myelin degradation with pronounced remyelination and protoplasmatic gliosis. Toluidine blue, x 1000. **e** Early stage of shadow plaque formation, lack of myelin degradation products; still pronounced protoplasmatic gliosis. Toluidine blue, x 1000. **f** Typical shadow plaque with protoplasmatic gliosis. Toluidine blue, x 1000

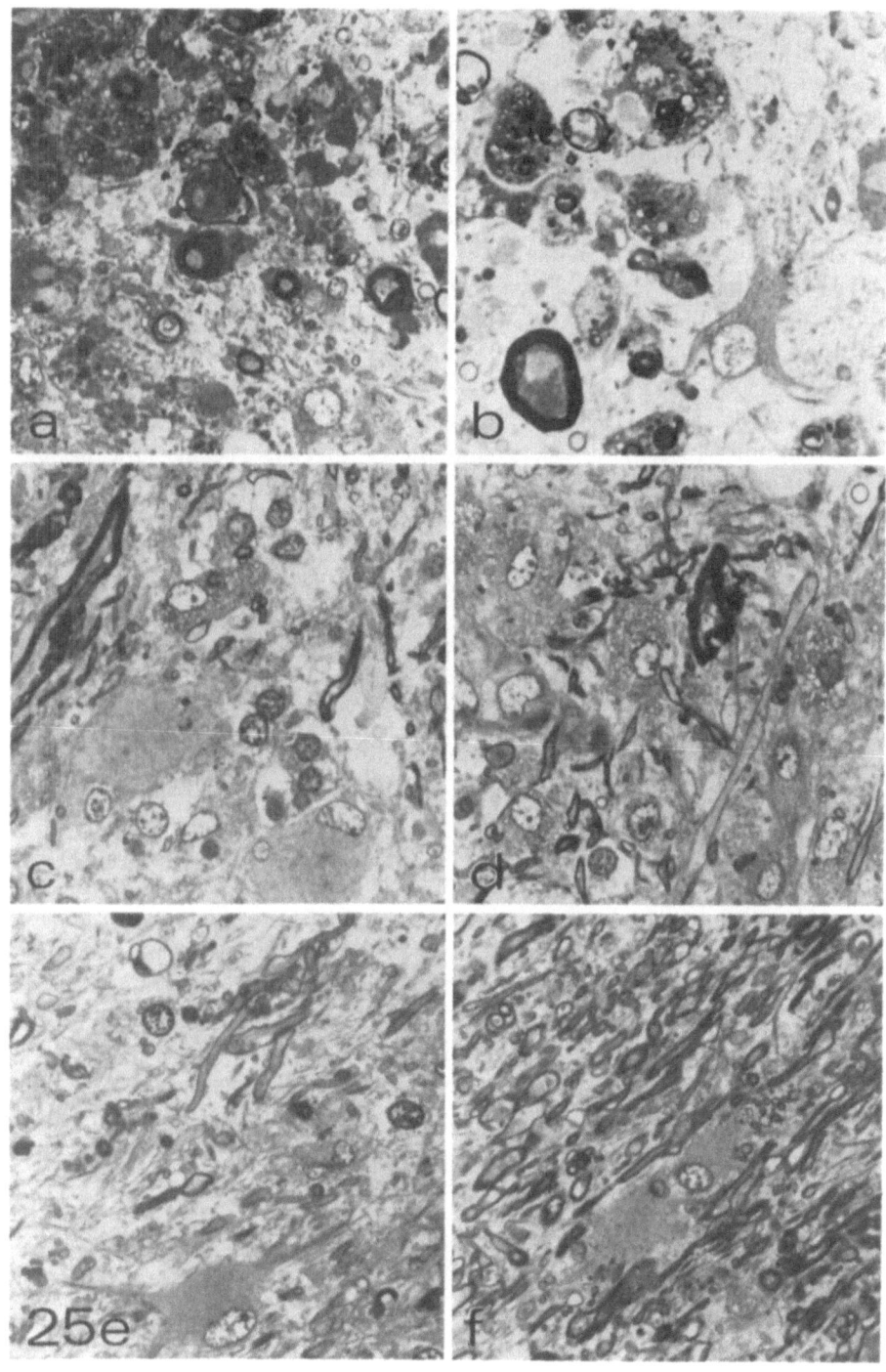

69

contain immunoglobulins (Dubois-Dalcq et al. 1975; Prineas and Raine 1976; Mussini et al. 1977). The uptake and degradation of serum proteins and tracers in astrocytes in diseases with blood-brain barrier damage are well documented in a large variety of different experimental models and human diseases (Brett and Weller 1978). Furthermore, especially intense accumulation of immunoglobulins in astrocytes but also in other cells of the brain (ependyma) has been noted in diseases with intrathecal immunoglobulin synthesis like MS and subacute sclerosing panencephalitis (Auff and Budka 1980). It has not yet been resolved, however, to what extent this diffuse imbibition of cells with immunoglobulins is due to a postmortem artifact facilitated by cell membrane autolysis (Auff and Budka 1980).

Therefore, comparing the structural features of MS lesions with those of chronic EAE lesions, it is evident that the patterns of gliosis are similar, provided that the early chronic stage is compared with acute MS and the late chronic stage with typical chronic MS. It is, however, still unknown what factors control the glia reaction in the individual plaque.

There are several possible explanations for the development of gliosis in EAE. One important factor is the extent of destruction of tissue components in the individual lesions. This may well explain the difference in extent of astroglia scar formation between plaques in the gray and white matter. Furthermore, extensive gliosis in periventricular plaques in EAE is generally preceded by secondary axonal destruction which is more extensive in these lesions than in plaques in other areas of the brain and spinal cord (Lassmann et al. 1980b). Another important factor in inducing gliosis is chronic edema (Jacob 1948; Reichhardt 1957; Adams 1977). In this connection it is interesting to note that the most intense and vigorous glial reaction is noted in destructive chronic EAE lesions, which are accompanied by massive vascular changes, the appearance of small venous thrombi, and small perivenous hemorrhages during the active stage of plaque formation. More difficult is the explanation of glia activation in the apparently normal white matter (Allen and McKeown 1979; Allen et al. 1979). In chronic inactive cases this finding may be to a large extent attributed to remyelination and repair of preexisting lesions. However, the presence of early stages of glia activation in the periplaque regions of actively demyelinating chronic lesions indicates that some pathogenetic factors (inflammatory mediators or liberated debris) themselves may activate astrocytes. Recently it has been shown in vitro that certain lymphokines may stimulate proliferation of

Fig. 26 a–h. Gliosis in chronic multiple sclerosis: same patient as described in Fig. 22. **a, b** Section ▷ through frontal white matter with numerous plaques in different stages; the lesions shown in **c–h** are labeled with *arrows;* note the absence of fibrillar gliosis in lesion in **c**. **a** Klüver, **b** Holzer, x 1. **c, d** Initial lesion with massive active demyelination and earliest myelin degradation products; note the intense protoplasmatic gliosis. **c** Klüver-Pas, x 300; **d** Toluidine blue, x 500. **e, f** Plaque in the sudanophilic stage of myelin degradation with the beginning of remyelination; protoplasmatic and the beginning of fibrillar gliosis. **e** H&E, x 300; **f** Toluidine blue, x500. **g, h** Typical shadow plaques with lack of myelin degradation products and fibrillary gliosis. **g** H&E, x 300; **h** Toluidine blue, x 500

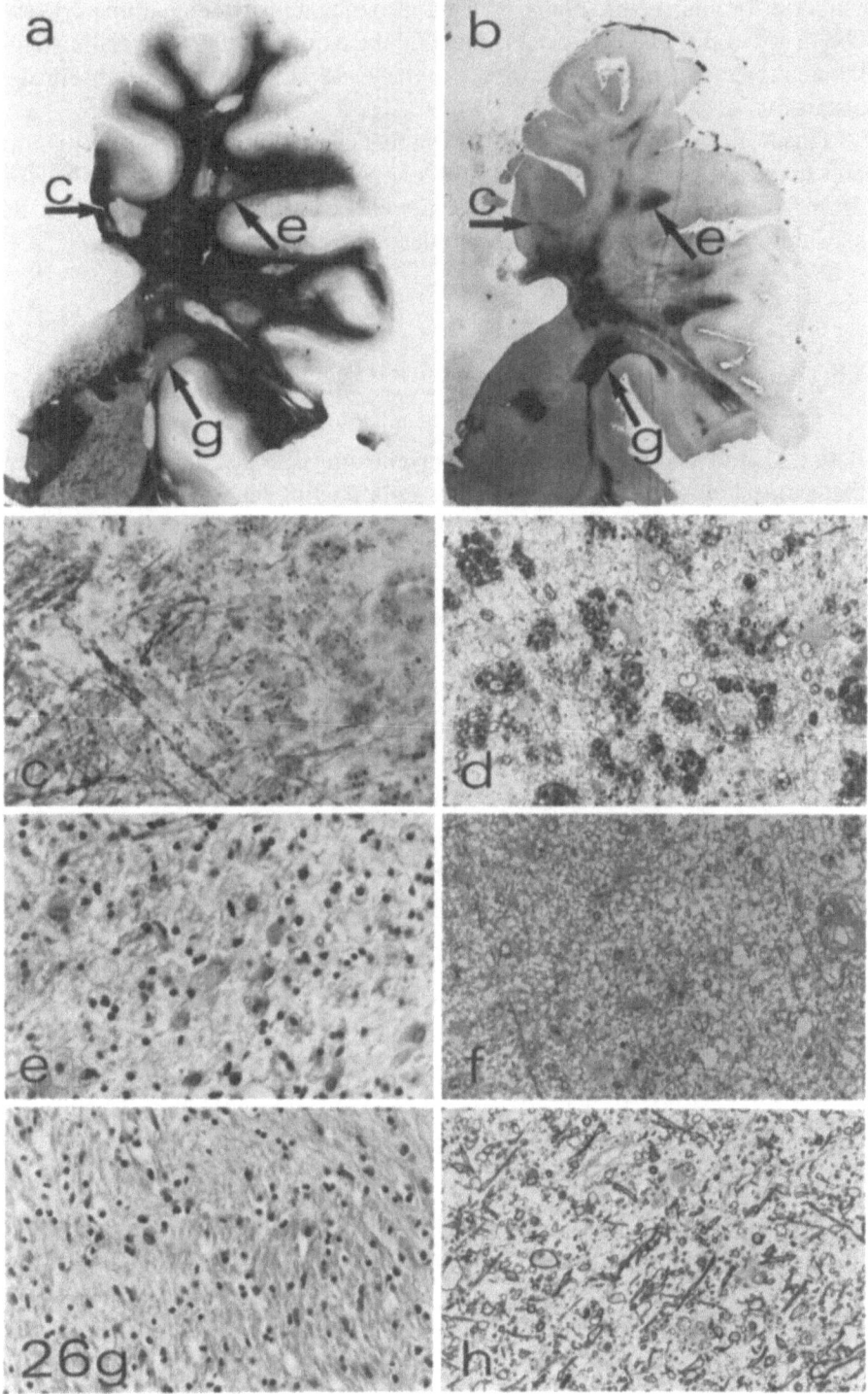

astrocytes (Fontana et al. 1980a, b). Thus also the intensity of inflammatory reaction in active as well as inactive plaques and the extent of cellular liberation of inflammatory mediators may contribute to the glial scar formation in demyelinated plaques.

Finally, it has not yet been clarified whether glia activation by itself may contribute to the pathogenesis of the lesions. McKeown and Allen (1978) described that the majoritiy of lysosomal enzymes which could be involved in destruction and degradation of myelin in MS plaques are derived from astrocytes.

4.8 Axonal and Neuronal Pathology

Both EAE and MS are inflammatory demyelinating diseases. This alone indicates that axonal and neuronal damage is not a dominating feature of the pathology.

It has been known since the earliest descriptions of the pathology of these diseases, however, that a reduction of axonal profiles in nearly all demyelinated lesions occurs, which may be sometimes extensive (Lumsden 1970). Furthermore, a large variety of nerve cell changes may be found in the brain and spinal cord lesions in MS patients and EAE animals which in general are interpreted as secondary alterations like central chromatolysis and ischemic-anoxic nerve cell damage. Occasionally, however, changes have been described, indicating a possible immunological attack against nerve cells in addition to primary demyelination.

4.8.1 Experimental Allergic Encephalomyelitis

In ordinary acute EAE destruction of neurons and axons was either not observed at all or was found in a few instances in perivascular demyelinated lesions (Morgan 1946; Wolf et al. 1947; Waksman and Adams 1962; Lampert 1965). In hyperacute lesions axonal damage is frequent (Levine and Wenk 1965; Levine et al. 1965; Lampert 1967) and even extreme in the EAE model of necrotic myelopathy (Levine and Sowinski 1976). All of these lesions have in common that axonal destruction correlates well with the overall destructiveness of the lesions, thus indicating that axonal destruction is a nonspecific consequence of inflammatory lesions in EAE (Waksman and Adams 1962).

In chronic EAE a similar pattern is observed. The more intense the inflammatory reaction during the stage of active demyelination the higher the degree of axonal destruction (Ferraro and Cazzullo 1948). Nerve cell changes in chronic EAE consist mainly of central chromatolysis (Fig. 27c) and sometimes "fatty degeneration" (Wolf et al. 1947). Axonal degeneration depends to some extent on the topographical localization of the lesion. Small caliber axons in periventricular plaques

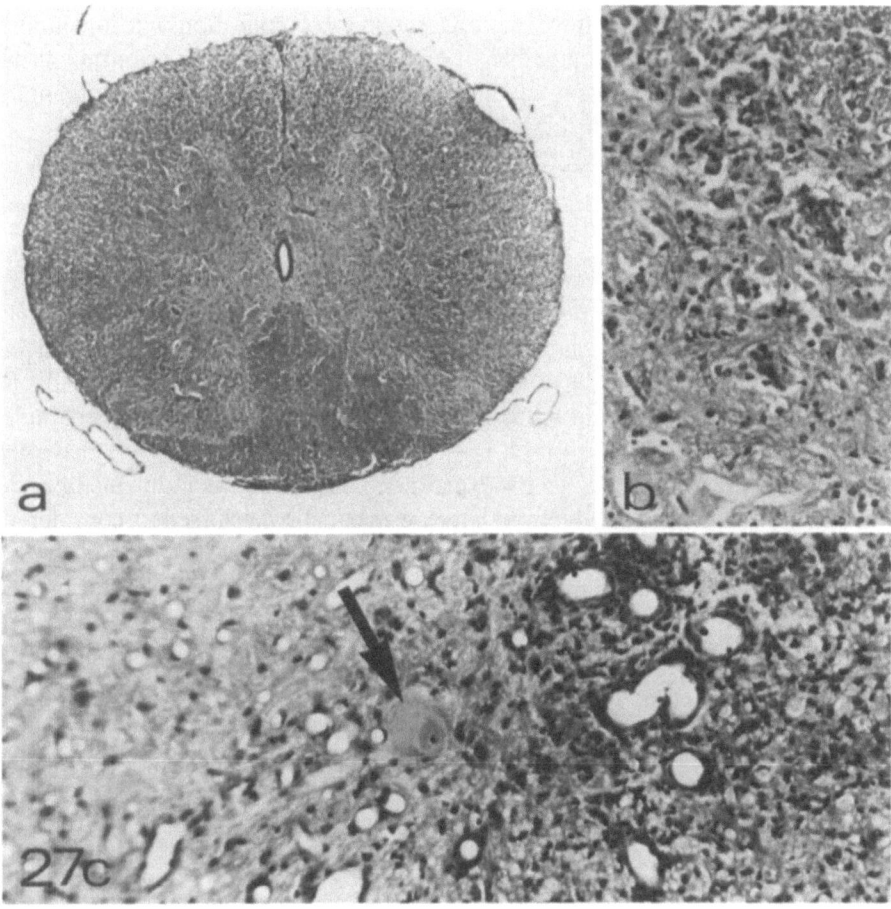

Fig. 27 a-c. Axonal and neuronal involvement in chronic relapsing EAE. **a** Animal with exceptionally, severe destruction of anterior horn cells in the early chronic stage of chronic relapsing EAE. H&E, x 25. **b** Higher magnification of **a**, showing inflammatory infiltrates and anterior horn cell destruction. H&E, x 300. **c** Central chromatolysis of anterior horn neuron adjacent to demyelinating EAE lesion *(arrow)*. H&E, x 700

and optic nerves are apparently more susceptible to damage compared with the large axons in spinal cord lesions (Lassmann et al. 1980b).

There seem to be few exceptions of the secondary involvement of axons and neurons in chronic EAE. In rare instances Jervis and Koprowski (1948) found areas where inflammatory cells surrounded nerve cells which seemed to undergo degenerative changes. In the corresponding figure typical alterations of neuronophagia are shown. In our experience in chronic relapsing EAE such lesions can be noted exceptionally, which in one animal in addition to the presence of demyelinated plaques showed a pathohistological pattern of extensive anterior horn destruction (Fig. 27a, b). Considering the rare incidence of this phenomenon it cannot be excluded that such a disease pattern is due to secondary complications like infections. Alternatively, however, it is possible that in these instances the immunological reaction is directed toward an antigen, which is equally present in myelin and neurons (like, e. g., GM_1-ganglioside).

4.8.2 Multiple Sclerosis

In multiple sclerosis the presence of axonal loss within demyelinated plaques and the ocurrence of secondary neuronal changes in the gray matter have been well known since the earliest descriptions of the pathology of this disease (Charcot 1868; Marburg 1906; Lumsden 1970). It is also well established that axonal loss is variable from plaque to plaque within different MS cases and also within one single case (Lumsden 1970).

Axonal loss in MS plaques seems to play an important role in inducing the residual functional deficit resulting from large demyelinating lesions. It is considered by most authors working on MS pathology that axonal loss is secondary to demyelination and dependent upon the intensity of the inflammatory reaction during the active phase of the lesion. However, similarly to in EAE, exceptional cases of active MS are described with a pattern of neuronal destruction comparable to neuronophagia in addition to the presence of demyelinated plaques (Fränkel and Jakob 1913). The significance of this finding in MS pathology is still unresolved.

4.9 Meningeal Pathology

The presence of meningeal pathology is frequently ignored in studies dealing with MS and EAE. This is surprising for several reasons. The blood-brain barrier in the meninges shows a higher permeability than that in the CNS parenchyma (Waksman 1960; Westergaard and Brightman 1973), and thus initial inflammation may be facilitated in meningeal vessels. In addition, the cerebrospinal fluid in MS as well as EAE contains a relatively high amount of immunoglobulins (Tourtellotte 1970; Link and Tibbling 1977; Mehta et al. 1981), which are at least partly synthesized from inflammatory cells in the meninges (Guseo and Jellinger 1975; Grundke-Iqbal et al. 1980). This is not only used for diagnosis but may also play a role in the pathogenesis of the lesions. Furthermore, the sink action of the CSF may be important in the removal of cells and debris from the lesions.

4.9.1 Experimental Allergic Encephalomyelitis

In acute EAE the meninges are generally the first target of inflammation (Waksman and Adams 1962). Meningeal inflammatory infiltrates may be noted as early

74

as 6 days after sensitization, at a stage preceding the onset of clinical disease for several days. Furthermore, in some "EAE-resistent" animals, inflammatory infiltrates following sensitization with CNS tissue or MBP may be found in the meninges in spite of the absence of inflammation in the parenchyma and of clinical disease of the animal. Initial stages of inflammation in the meninges can be noted around small meningeal venoles at the area of anastomosis between meningeal and parenchymal venoles (Lassmann et al. 1981b). These areas have been shown in tracer studies to have a relatively higher permeability for the exchange of proteins from the circulation into the CSF and vice versa (Lassmann, unpublished). Later during the development of the disease (during the first days after clinical onset of acute EAE) meningeal infiltrates spread out and become more diffuse. At this stage generally a pronounced exchange of cells (large mononuclear cells and phagocytes) through the glia limitans between the CNS parenchyma and the CSF can be found. Meningeal inflammation may persist for considerable time after recovery of animals from EAE (at least several months), in animals which show no clinical evidence for ongoing chronic disease.

In chronic EAE, initial stages of plaque formation in a relapse generally show meningeal changes similar to those which can be found in the early stages of acute EAE. However, with the development of large demyelinated plaques, inflammatory changes in the meninges are not generalized but restricted to an area exactly covering the underlying demyelinated plaques (Lassmann et al. 1981b). In this location the inflammatory reaction is much more pronounced than in acute EAE, with massive perivenous accumulation of lymphocytes and plasma cells and extensive infiltration by debris-containing phagocytes. When debris is removed and the lesions are inactive, the inflammatory reaction in the overlying meninges decreases and is replaced by pronounced fibrosis and thickening of the pia mater. In these lesions connections of meningeal fibroblasts with the cell processes of the glia limitans may frequently be found (Raine et al. 1978b; Lassmann et al. 1981b). Fibrosis of the meninges is also found in the area of the dural sinus in the chronic stage of EAE. It is at present not clear whether these structural changes in the sinus may affect the resorption of CSF from the CNS compartment. It must be noted, however, that a moderate degree of communicating hydrocephalus is frequent in chronic EAE animals.

The choroid plexus is also a frequent target of inflammation in EAE. During chronic EAE choroid plexus inflammation is present to a variable degree in nearly all animals investigated, regardless of their clinical disease state (acute exacerbation or remission). It is of interest that in the choroid plexus accumulation of lymphatic tissue may sometimes be found in chronic EAE comparable to secondary lymph follicles in organs other than the brain.

Another interesting aspect of choroid plexus pathology in chronic relapsing EAE is the frequent but not regular presence of PAS-positive amorphous perivascular deposits, which by immunofluorescence can be identified as accumulations of immunoglobulin and complement (Grundke-Iqbal et al. 1980). It is at present not clear whether these deposits of immune complexes in the choroid plexus are pathogenetically relevant.

4.9.2 Multiple Sclerosis

Inflammation in the meninges of the CNS of MS patients has been well known since the early descriptions of the disease (Marburg 1906; Guseo and Jellinger 1975). This seeding of inflammatory cells in the meninges seems to be responsible for the moderate increase of cells in the CSF of MS patients. Furthermore, the occurrence of plasma cells in the infilrates (Guseo and Jellinger 1975) may partially be the source of immunoglobulins in the CSF, which are a characteristic feature of chronic MS. In a detailed study of inflammatory reaction in MS, Guseo and Jellinger (1975) observed an incidence of meningeal inflammation in 41% of all investigated cases, and meningeal inflammation was more pronounced and frequent in cases with active demyelination. The incidence of meningeal inflammation of 41% in MS cases is surprisingly low and probably related to the extent of sampling of tissue blocks in MS cases. However, the overall intensity of meningeal inflammation is more pronounced in EAE than in MS.

Focal alterations can be seen in the meninges of MS patients in areas where plaques reach the outer surface of the spinal cord. In these lesions a transfer of inflammatory cells through the glia limitans is observed leading to accumulation of lipid-containing phagocytes in the pia mater in actively demyelinating plaques. Thus, similarly to in chronic relapsing EAE, the meninges seem to be an important source for inflammatory cells and mediators during initiation of plaque formation and seem to play a role in debris removal during the clearing stage of a plaque (Marburg 1906). In chronic inactive plaques, which reach to the outer surface of CNS tissue, irregularities in the glia limitans together with adhesions and connections of astrocytes and meningeal cells were frequently observed (Marburg 1906). It is interesting to note that also in MS these meningeal alterations are not diffusely distributed in the pia but strictly localized at the surface extension of the demyelinated lesion (Marburg 1906).

4.10 Peripheral Nervous System Pathology

One of the major differences between experimental allergic encephalomyelitis and multiple sclerosis is believed to be in the pathological alterations in the peripheral nervous system. Whereas in EAE, inflammatory demyelinating lesions in the PNS are frequent following sensitization with central nervous systems antigens, MS is generally believed to be an exclusive CNS disease. However, reviewing the literature dealing with EAE, it becomes evident that the incidence and extent of PNS involvement are variable, depending on the strain of animals used in the experiments and on the antigen used for sensitization (Alvord 1970).

In multiple sclerosis some cases of indisputable inflammatory demyelination in the peripheral nerves and roots have been described (Henschen 1896; Strähuber 1903; Dinkler 1904; Marburg 1906; Schob 1923; Pette 1928; Ketelaer et al. 1966; Ninfo et al. 1967; Jellinger 1969; Schoene et al. 1977; Van Gehuchten et al. 1966; Pollock et al. 1977; Lassmann et al. 1981d), although the incidence of PNS involvement in MS seems to be very low (Jellinger 1969).

4.10.1 PNS Involvement in Different Models of Chronic EAE

When different models of chronic EAE are compared with each other it is interesting to note that in spite of nearly identical sensitization procedures the incidence of demyelinating lesions in the PNS may be extremely variable. The spectrum ranges from low incidence (10% in Hartley guinea pigs, Himberg, Austria) to higher frequencies in strain 13 animals (75%, Madrid and Wisniewski 1978) to models in rats and rabbits of predominant PNS disease in the chronic stage with only a few or absent CNS lesions (Prineas et al. 1969; Lassmann et al. 1980a). Furthermore, the onset of PNS demyelination may be variable from model to model. In strain 13 guinea pigs substantial PNS demyelination was noted not earlier than 60–90 days after sensitization (Madrid and Wisniewski 1978), whereas in Hartley guinea pigs active PNS demyelination, if present at all, was found mainly during the subacute and early chronic stage of the disease (30–50 days after sensitization).

PNS lesions in chronic relapsing EAE are generally localized in the spinal roots with the highest incidence in the cauda equina followed by the trigeminal roots (Fig. 28). Large peripheral nerve trunks (sciatic or median nerve) are only exceptionally involved. The pattern of demyelination is described in detail in earlier studies (Wisniewski et al. 1969; Raine et al 1969; Madrid and Wisniewski 1978) and follows the pattern observed in experimental allergic neuritis induced by sensitization with PNS tissue (Lampert 1969; Pollard et al. 1975). The simultaneous presence of active demyelination and reparatory changes of peripheral nerve fibers indicates the chronic (recurrent?) nature of PNS demyelination in chronic EAE (Madrid and Wisniewski 1978) (Fig. 28e, f).

The involvement of the peripheral nervous system in experimental allergic encephalomyelitis is not surprising as several antigens which seem to be pathogenetically relevant (myelin basic protein, galactocerebroside and ganglioside) are shared between the central and peripheral myelin; and an immune response against these antigens may elicit demyelination in the CNS or PNS in vivo and in vitro (Nagai et al. 1976; London 1971; Greenfield et al. 1973; Saida et al. 1978a, 1979b; Dubois-Dalqu et al. 1970). The low incidence of PNS involvement in some models of chronic EAE, however, indicates that other antigens restricted to CNS myelin or oligodendroglia cell membrane may be pathogenetically relevant for the disease.

4.10.2 Peripheral Nervous System Involvement in Multiple Sclerosis

Alterations in the peripheral nervous system (PNS) in multiple sclerosis have been frequently found; however, most of these changes can be explained as secondary nerve damage due to malnutrition, vitamin deficiency, etc. (Hasson et al. 1958). On the other hand, several studies have documented the presence of primary, inflammatory demyelinating lesions in exceptional MS cases. Similarly to in chronic EAE, PNS demyelination has been noted mainly in the spinal roots (Fig. 28g); the spectrum of alterations in the roots included inflammation (Pette 1928; Ninfo et al. 1967; Lassmann et al. 1981d), primary demyelination (Dinkler 1904; Marburg 1906; Pollock et al. 1977; Lassmann et al. 1981d), plaque-like distribution of demyelinated lesions (Van Gehuchten 1966; Lassmann et al. 1981d), remyelination (Pollock et al. 1977; Lassmann et al. 1981d), and the formation of onion bulbs (Dinkler 1904; Schob 1923; Jellinger 1969). The incidence of demyelinating lesions in the PNS in typical chronic MS seems to be very low, and has been calculated by Jellinger (1969) at one out of 70 investigated cases. However, PNS involvement in acute MS is frequent (two out of three cases, Marburg 1906; three out of three cases, Pette 1928; two out of six cases, own material). Although the case numbers are too small for the determination of an exact incidence, this possible PNS involvement in acute MS must be kept in mind as it may obscure the clinical diagnosis. Furthermore, CNS involvement with perivenous inflammation and demyelination has been noted in the Landry-Guillain-Barré syndrome (Polan and Baker 1942; Baker 1943). In a series of 50 cases of inflammatory polyradiculitis, Haymaker and Kernohan (1949) described ten cases with CNS involvement. Further immunological studies are necessary to determine the pathogenetic factors responsible for the cross reaction between CNS and PNS myelin in human diseases.

4.11 Patterns of Plaque Growth

Much attention has been paid in multiple sclerosis pathology to the mechanisms involved in the enlargement of the lesions. There are mainly two different views of how large demyelinated plaques in MS develop. On the one hand, large lesions

---

Fig. 28 a–g. PNS involvement in chronic relapsing EAE and MS. **a, b** Sprague Dawley rat with chronic relapsing EAE, 60 dps; predominantly inflammatory type of PNS pathology with little demyelination. **a** H&E; **b** Klüver, x 30. **c, d** Sprague Dawley rat with chronic EAE, 63 dps; trigeminal ganglion; large plaque-like demyelinating lesion. **c** H&E; **d** Klüver, x 30. **e, f** Sprague Dawley rat with chronic EAE 45 dps; demyelinating lesion in the cauda equina with active demyelination and remyelination. **e** Toluidine blue, x 80; **f** Toluidine blue, x 1000. **g** Cervical root of a patient with acute MS (Lassmann et al. 1981d). Plaque-like, segmental demyelination in the root. Toluidine blue, x 80

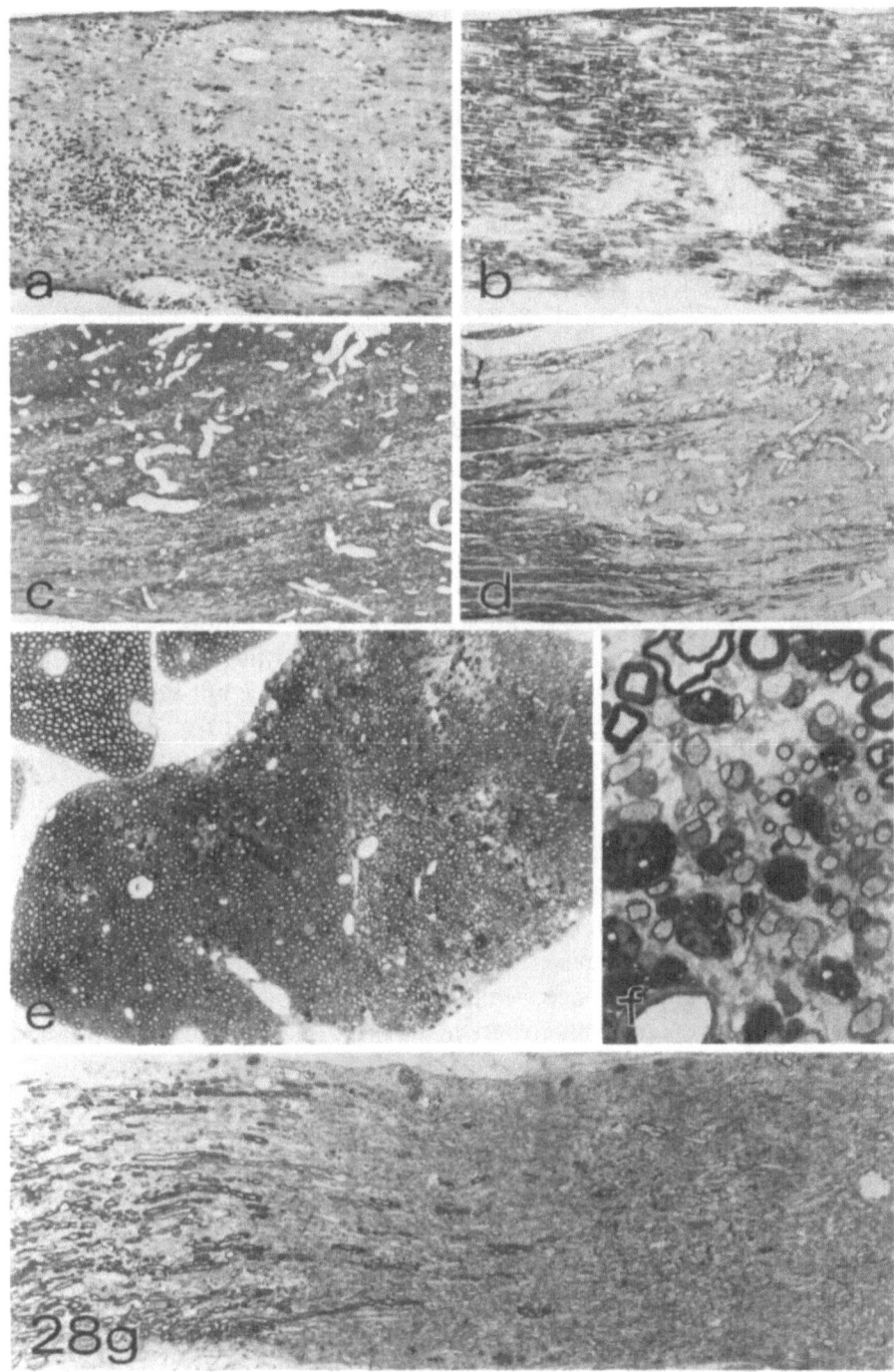

may be formed by the confluence of multiple small perivenous rims of demyelination (Marburg 1906; Dawson 1916). On the other hand, plaques may originate from radial extension of a small perivenous lesion, which enlarges by active demyelination on its circumference (Hallervorden 1940; Steiner 1931). Although present evidence from MS pathology suggests that both types of plaque growth may occur, there is still some controversy as to which type is the more frequent and important.

One major difference between MS and EAE pathology was believed to lie in the mechanisms of lesional growth (Alvord et al. 1979). The occurence of confluence of perivenous active lesions in EAE has been well known since the earliest descriptions of this disease (Rivers et al. 1933; Ferraro and Cazzullo 1948; Wolf et al. 1947); however, radial plaque growth was believed to be absent in EAE lesions (Alvord et al. 1979). These observations, however, were mainly based on the study of acute and subacute EAE.

4.11.1 Plaque Growth in Chronic EAE

In chronic relapsing EAE four different patterns of lesional growth can be found:

The *perivenous confluent plaque* is the most frequent type present in the central nervous system of chronic EAE animals (Figs. 20a, 30d). It is initiated by active perivenous demyelination (Fig. 30c, d). The perivenous rims of demyelination gradually enlarge and fuse with each other. This results in the formation of a large demyelinated plaque with characteristic finger-like perivenous extensions at its periphery. This type of lesion may be found at any stage of chronic relapsing EAE; it is, however, more frequent in the subacute and early chronic stages than in the late chronic stage of the disease.

The second type is the *rapidly developing plaque* (Fig. 29b). It is found mainly in animals with a clear-cut relapsing disease pattern which suffer from a severe relapse of the disease after a prolonged remission period. In principle this plaque type is similar to the perivenous confluent lesion; the speed of demyelination, however, is so high that the perivenous pattern of the lesion can be recognized only during the 1st day after onset of the relapse. In later stages a large demyelinated lesion is formed which contains phagocytes uniformly scattered throughout the whole plaque which are loaded with myelin debris, all in the same stage of myelin degradation.

The third type is the *radial growth of a preexisting lesion* (Fig. 29c). This type is found mainly in the late chronic stage of the disease and especially in animals with a chronic progressive disease course. The center of these lesions is a demyelinated sclerotic plaque which is surrounded by zones of active demyelination either on the entire circumference or in small focal areas at the borders. Radial plaque growth at the entire circumference of the lesion is rare in chronic EAE. This is due mainly to anatomical reasons as the white matter is very small in guinea pigs, and

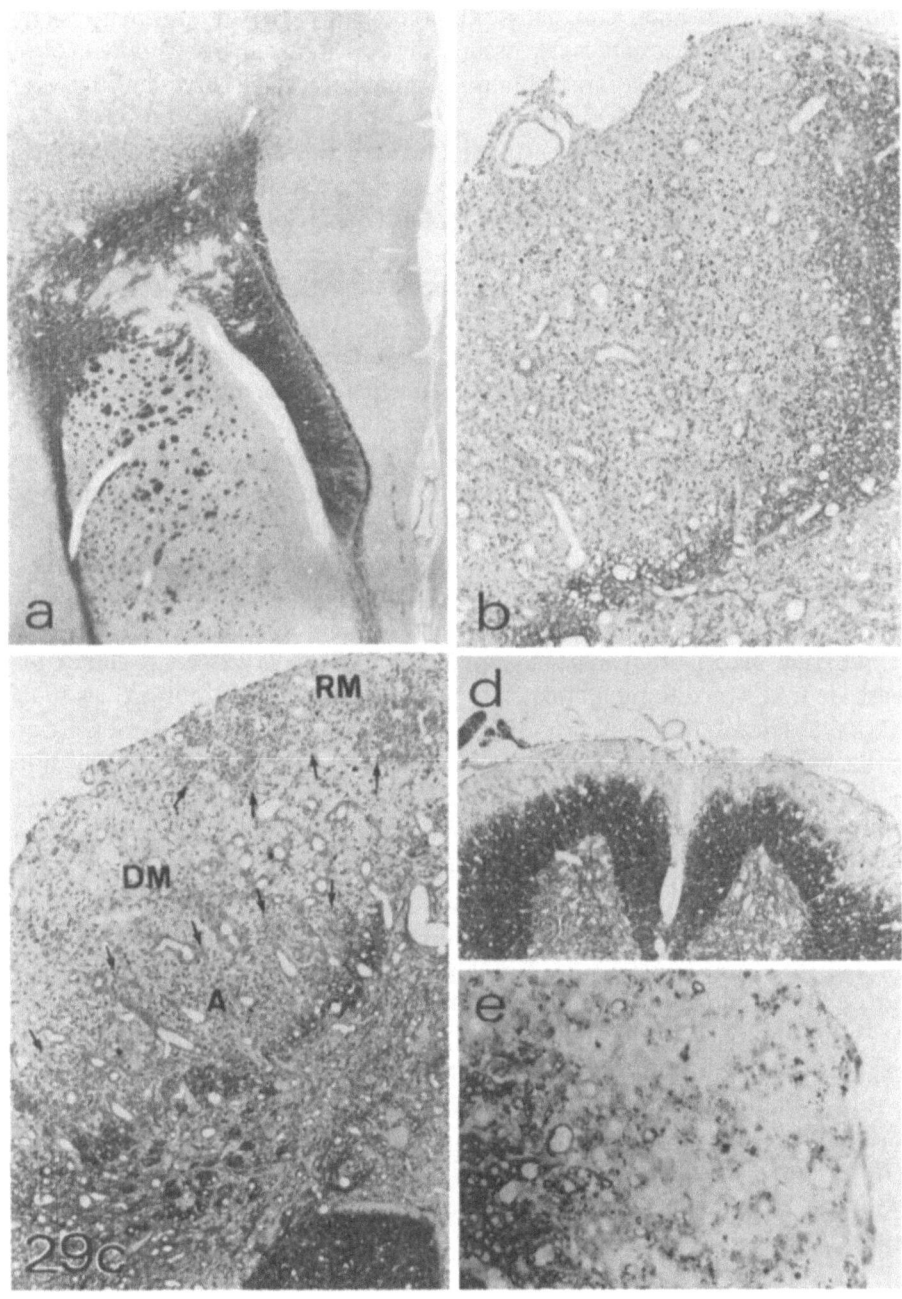

Fig. 29 a–e. Patterns of plaque growth in chronic relapsing EAE in guinea pigs. **a** Confluent perivenous lesions. Klüver, × 16. **b** Rapidly developing lesion; earliest stages of myelin debris are scattered throughout the whole lesion. Klüver, × 80. **c** Radial plaque growth; three lesion zones are visible (separated by *arrows*); *RM*, remyelinated zone; *DM*, demyelinated inactive zone; *A*, actively demyelinating zone. Klüver, × 50. **d, e** Cerebrospinal fluid oriented lesion. **d** Klüver, × 40; **e** Klüver, × 250

thus the borders of larger demyelinated lesions rapidly reach the gray matter or the outer and inner surface of the CNS tissue. However, focal radial enlargement of demyelinating lesions is a common finding in animals sampled later than 50 days after sensitization.

The fourth type of plaque growth is found in the *cerebrospinal fluid oriented lesions* (Fig. 29d, e). It is similar to the above-described radial plaque growth. It is characterized by a periventricular or subpial zone of demyelination which enlarges into the brain or spinal cord parenchyma by an active zone of demyelination. Similarly to the radially expanding lesions in the depth of the CNS tissue, this lesional type is found mainly in animals in the late chronic stage of chronic relapsing EAE.

In all four types of plaques the topographical relation to inflammatory infiltrates in the CNS can be established. Whereas in the first two the inflammatory cells are more evenly distributed around large drainage veins, small veins, and venoles, in plaques with radial growth inflammatory cuffs are generally found around large drainage veins or in the meninges. In the periventricular lesions the inflammatory cells on the ventricular surface (supraependymal cells) may also play a role in the pathogenesis of lesion formation (Lassmann et al. 1981a).

In chronic relapsing EAE the size of the demyelinated lesions depends mainly upon the interval between sensitization and plaque formation (Lassmann et al. 1980b) (Fig. 30c, f). This can be best studied when animals with active clinical disease are studied at different time points after challenge. Hartley guinea pigs 10–20 days after sensitization show no or minimal demyelination in spite of extensive perivenous inflammation. During the subacute stage of the disease (20–40 days after sensitization) multiple perivenous rims of demyelination can be found in animals with active disease; however, confluence of perivenous lesions is generally absent. The earliest confluent demyelinated plaque in chronic EAE was noted 32 days after sensitization. In the majority of the animals, however, confluent lesions are noted not earlier than 40–50 days after sensitization. With increasing time after sensitization the plaque size enlarged, reaching maximal levels at 60–150 dps. It is interesting that in animals with chronic progressive EAE the size of individual plaques at a given time after sensitization is similar to that found in guinea pigs with chronic relapsing disease. As during the remission period active demyelination is sparse or absent in the spinal cord of animals with relapsing disease (Lassmann and Wisniewski 1978) the speed of demyelination must be higher than in chronic progressive lesions. This view is also supported by the observation that the above-described rapidly developing plaques are found mainly in animals with clear-cut relapsing EAE.

Fig. 30 a–f. Types of demyelinating lesions in acute and chronic EAE. **a, b** Demyelinated plaques in the ▷ periventricular white matter. x 3. **c** Typical perivenous demyelinating lesion of subacute EAE. Klüver, x 20. **d** Typical demyelinated plaques of chronic EAE, Klüver, x 20. **e** Cerebrospinal fluid oriented lesion, covering the entire circumference of the spinal cord. Klüver, x 20. **f** Nearly complete demyelination of a spinal cord segment. Klüver, x 20

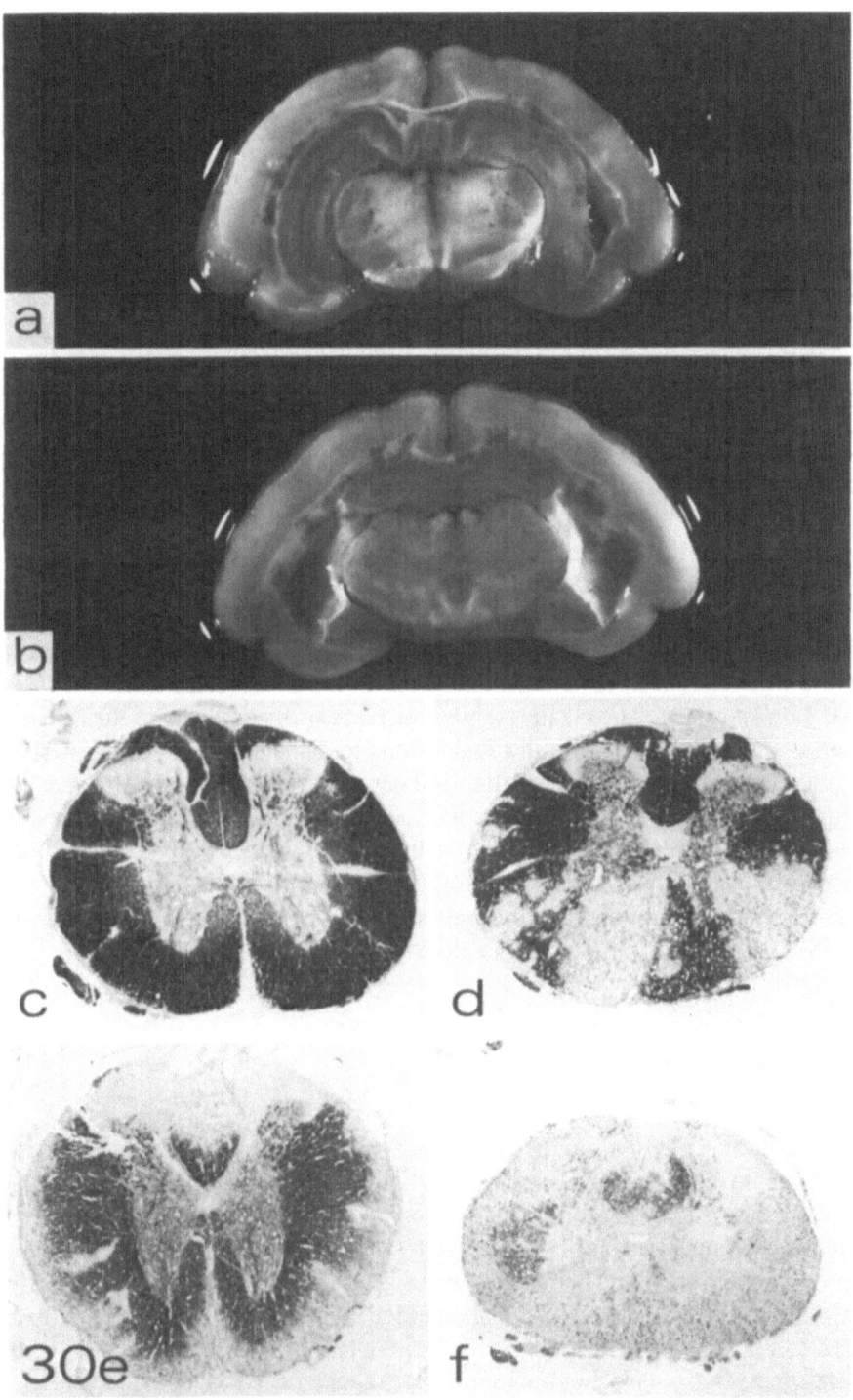

4.11.2 Mechanisms of Plaque Growth in Multiple Sclerosis

In multiple sclerosis similar mechanisms of plaque growth have been described in detail (Marburg 1906; Dawson 1916; Pette 1928; Steiner 1931; Hallervorden 1940; Lumsden 1970). In cases of acute MS the main type found was the confluence of adjacent perivenous lesions (Marburg 1906; Dawson 1916). Similarly synchronous demyelination in large plaques, as found in rapidly developing lesions in chronic relapsing EAE, is found mainly in cases of acute MS. These rapidly developing lesions can best be identified when the earliest myelin degradation products (positive in myelin stains like Luxol fast blue and Marchi reaction) are present in all the phagocytes which are scattered throughout the whole plaque.

Radial plaque growth of large lesions in the depth of the white matter or related to the inner and outer surface of the CNS is generally found in active cases of chronic MS (Steiner 1931, Pette 1928). It must be emphasized, however, that confluent perivenous lesions may also occur in chronic MS, whereas radial plaque growth is also found in acute MS cases.

Regarding the size of demyelinating lesions in humans a principally similar pattern to that in EAE is observed when inflammatory demyelinating diseases are regarded as a closely related group of disorders. Acute perivenous leukoencephalitis is accompanied by small perivenous rims of demyelination. The lesions in acute MS are in general still much smaller than typical chronic MS plaques. In contrast to EAE, however, in MS the plaques tend to increase with chronicity of the disease, whereas in EAE the size of individual lesions remains constant during the late chronic stage of the disease (later than 100 days after sensitization). This may be partly explained by anatomical differences, as the small size of the white matter in rodents limits firther extension of demyelinating lesions. However, even in areas where further growth of plaques is possible, in EAE animals no enlargement of plaques is found. This indicates that the pathogenetic events leading to demyelination in MS are active for longer periods than with chronic relapsing EAE.

4.12 Lesional Topography in the CNS

The destribution of lesions in the central nervous system is a feature of human inflammatory demyelinating diseases which has puzzled neuropathologists for many years. Lesions may be formed at any region of the CNS, and the localization of lesions is unpredictable. However, at least in chronic diseases like multiple sclerosis some areas of the brain and spinal cord are more frequently affected than others (Steiner 1931; Pette 1928; Hallervorden 1940; Fog 1950; Lumsden 1970; Oppenheimer 1978; Field 1979). In chronic relapsing EAE similar predilection sites of demyelinated plaques are found (Lassmann and Wisniewski 1979a; Lassmann et al. 1981a, b). Thus, a detailed analysis of structural events preceding the formation of lesions and occurring during plaque growth in this animal model may help to understand the peculiar lesional distribution in human inflammatory demyelinating diseases.

4.12.1 Lesional Distribution in EAE

In acute EAE (10–20 dps) the distribution of lesions is generally disseminated throughout the neuraxis. This is especially the case in highly susceptible animals with severe disease course and high mortality in acute EAE. The lesions are dominated by perivenous inflammation and small rims of demyelination surrounding veins of all sizes including small postcapillary venoles (Fig. 30c). The intensity of perivenous inflammation and demyelination is variable in different areas of the CNS. This can be best visualized in animals with mild or moderate disease severity. In these animals lesions are most frequently found in the lumbosacral portions of the spinal cord and in the fornix at the insertion of the choroid plexus.

In the chronic stage of chronic relapsing EAE the pattern of lesional distribution changes. Large demyelinated plaques, characteristic for the chronic stage of the disease, are either related to inflammatory infiltrates around large drainage veins or are oriented toward the inner and outer surface of the CNS. They are frequently located in a symmetrical position in the periventricular white matter and in the spinal cord (Lassmann et al. 1981a, b) (Fig. 30).

The lesional incidence in the brain and spinal cord in chronic relapsing EAE has already been described in detail (Lassmann and Wisniewski 1979c). The highest lesional density is found in the thoracic spinal cord, followed by, in order of incidence, the cervical spinal cord, centrum semiovale, lumbosacral spinal cord, optic nerve, fornix, and cerebellar white matter. Large lesions in the brain stem in chronic EAE animals are rare because of the high mortality of animals with even small perivenous lesions in this location. It must be noted, however, that the incidence of lesions in the brain versus the spinal cord may be different when different strains of animals are used for the experiments. In the strain of Hartley guinea pigs (Himberg, Austria) used by us at present, the incidence of periventricular demyelinated plaques is much higher than in the results described above (Fig. 30a, b). Furthermore, when Sprague Dawley rats are sensitized for chronic relapsing EAE, lesions within the CNS are most pronounced in the spinal cord and the cerebellar white matter (Lassmann et al. 1980a (Fig. 31). A similar predilection for lesions in the lower portions of the spinal cord and cerebellum in rats has already been noted by Levine et al. (1967). The lumbosacral spinal cord, the region most frequently affected in acute EAE, shows only a low lesional incidence and small lesions in the chronic stage of EAE. This is especially surprising as the distribution of large drainage veins in the thoracic and lumbosacral spinal cord is essentially similar. As most veins and venules in the lower portions of the cord show some degree of fibrosis in animals sampled after the acute episode, a mechanisms similar to that described as vascular

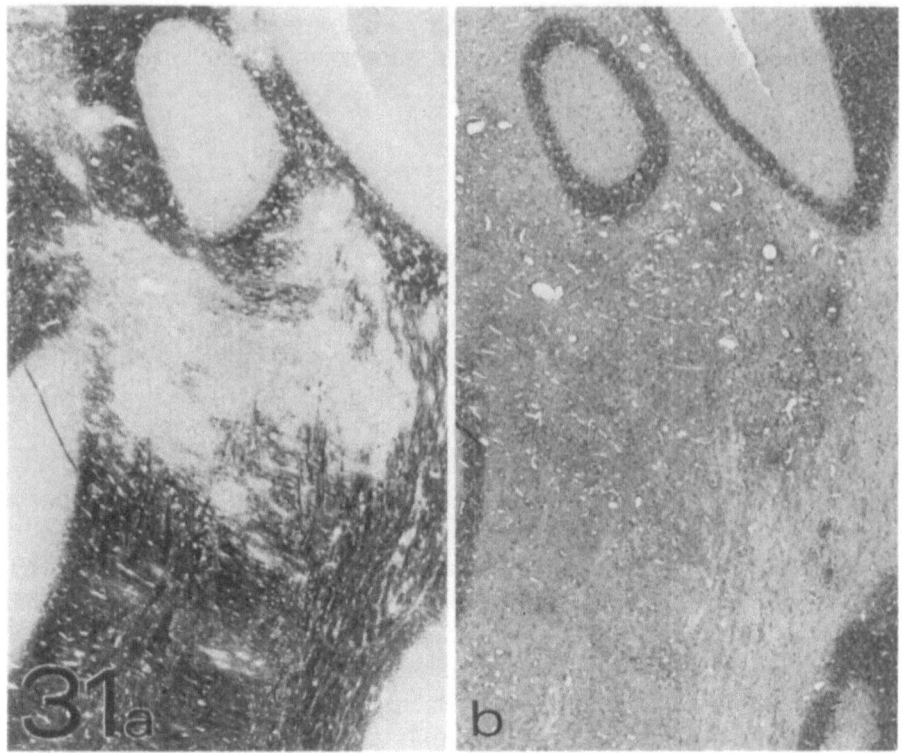

Fig. 31 a, b. Chronic EAE in Sprague Dawley rats. **a, b** Large confluent demyelinated plaque in the cerebellar white matter. **a** Klüver; **b** PTAH, x 50

blockade in EAE by Levine (1970), may be responsible for the low lesional incidence in this region in the chronic stage of the disease.

It is interesting that in chronic relapsing EAE there is an inverse relationship between the severity and size of lesions in the brain and those in the spinal cord. Animals with massive, large lesions in the spinal cord in general have a low lesional incidence in the brain and vice versa.

It is not known at present what factors regulate the appearance of lesions in a given topographical localization. One important factor controlling lesional topography is the density of veins in the tissue. Thus areas with a high density of large drainage veins are more susceptible to the formation of demyelinated plaques than others (Waksman 1960b; Lassmann et al. 1981b). However, this does not explain why other regions with a similar venous density are spared in the same animals. Thus, other local factors like the mechanical strain of the tissue, as discussed for spinal cord lesions in MS (Oppenheimer 1978), may be of additional importance for lesional distribution.

During the early chronic stage of chronic relapsing EAE (40–100 dps), the perivenous distribution of lesions can be easily identified. The lesions are formed by confluence of small perivenous rims of demyelination and then grow further by radial extension of preexisting plaques. However, especially in later stages after sensitization another lesional type is frequently noted. This type is clearly oriented toward the inner and outer surface of the CNS, resulting in a rim of demyelination evenly surrounding the spinal cord surface (Fig. 30e) or following the ependymal lining in the cerebral hemispheres. This type of lesion closely resembles the *Mantelherde* in multiple sclerosis. In the spinal cord this lesional type may be easily explained as it is always combined with meningeal inflammation on the entire spinal cord circumference (Lassmann et al. 1981b). Similarly the majority of periventricular lesions can be traced to the inflammatory cuffs around the large drainage veins which fuse with the vena cerebri magna of Galen. Furthermore, the increased numbers of supraependymal inflammatory cells on the surface of periventricular lesions may represent a reservoir of pathogenetic factors leading to demyelination (Lassmann et al. 1981a). An additional pathogenetic aspect may be that the moderate dilatation of the ventricles frequently observed in chronic EAE animals may alter the permeability of subependymal venules and veins (Lassmann et al. 1981a).

In summary, there are still many questions unresolved regarding the pathogenetic factors leading to the precipitation of a lesion in a given place of the CNS. There are, however, two main events governing the lesional distribution in EAE:
– The diffuse, sleeve-like distribution of demyelination in acute EAE which surrounds all venous segments including small postcapillary venules changes into a more focal distribution of demyelinated plaques in chronic EAE oriented toward large drainage veins or toward the inner and outer surface of the CNS. This difference is responsible for the high incidence of chronic EAE lesions in areas with a high density of large drainage veins (Lassmann et al. 1981a, b).
– All active chronic EAE lesions are oriented toward areas with seeding of inflammatory cells (lymphocytes and plasma cells) in the CNS. This seeding of inflammatory cells is found in the Virchow-Robin spaces of large drainage veins and in the connective tissue of the meninges and choroid plexus.

4.12.2 Lesional Topography in Human Inflammatory Demyelinating Diseases

In human inflammatory demyelinating diseases the pattern of demyelination and lesional distribution varies in a similar way during chronicity of the disease as previously described in EAE (Seitelberger 1967, 1973). In acute perivenous leukoencephalitis perivenous inflammatory infiltrates and perivenous sleeves of demyelination are disseminated and may be found at any location in the CNS. They involve all types of veins including the smallest ramifications. On the contrary in chronic MS demyelinated plaques are focal, oriented toward larger vessels, and localized mainly in certain predilection sites in the CNS (Seitelberger 1967, 1973). This different pattern can be best studied in cases of acute MS where typical lesions of acute perivenous leukoencephalitis and chronic MS can be found in close vicinity.

In chronic MS the relationship of large demyelinated plaques to the distribution of large veins is clearly established (Rindfleisch 1863; Dawson 1916; Siemerling and Raeke 1914; Lumsden 1970; Field 1979), and is especially well documented in the spinal cord (Fog 1950). Although the lesions are generally found in areas of high density of drainage veins (Fog 1950), not all drainage veins are the center of demyelinated lesions. Thus, other factors, e. g., the mechanical strain on the vasculature may help to precipitate a lesion at a given place (Oppenheimer 1978). In addition to these lesions oriented toward veins, there is another plaque type in chronic MS which is related to the inner and outer surfaces of the CNS (Steiner 1931; Pette 1928; Hallervorden 1940). The most classical lesion of this type is the so-called *Mantelherd* in chronic MS (Steiner 1931). This orientation of lesions toward the inner and outer surface of the CNS has led to the concept that demyelinating factors may enter the brain via the cerebrospinal fluid. However, not much attention was paid in these studies to the distribution of inflammatory infiltrates in the CSF-oriented lesions. In the spinal cord Marburg (1906) described in detail that in active surface-oriented lesions the meninges are heavily infiltrated by inflammatory cells in an area covering the surface extension of the plaque. Furthermore, exchange of inflammatory cells through the glia limitans between the meninges and the spinal cord parenchyma was noted (Marburg 1906). Thus, at least in the spinal cord the CSF-oriented lesions are also strictly related to the seeding of inflammatory cells.

Lesions in MS may appear everywhere in the brain and spinal cord (Lumsden 1970). There are, however, some predilection points for lesion formation: especially the lateral angle of the lateral ventricles (*Wetterwinkel*; Steiner 1931), the cerebellar peduncles (Field 1979), the corticosubcortical areas (Lumsden 1970), the lateral surface of the spinal cord (Fog 1950; Oppenheimer 1978), and the optic nerves. The periventricular plaques in MS are so characteristic that Hallervorden (1940) doubted the diagnosis of MS in cases with absent periventricular demyelination. However, in acute MS (Marburg's type) periventricular lesions are rare and if present are small and frequently not related to the ventricular surface. Instead there is a very high incidence of demyelinated plaques in the brain stem, especially in the pons and the medulla. The high incidence of brain stem lesions in cases of acute MS may be due to a selection mechanism, as the mortality of patients with large brain stem plaques is higher than that found in patients with lesions elsewhere in the brain or spinal cord. It is, however, interesting to note that in these acute MS cases the predilection sites for lesions in typical chronic MS are apparently not more frequently involved than other regions of the brain. This is similar to our observation in the early chronic phase of chronic relapsing EAE, where lesions are more randomly distributed in the CNS than those found in late chronic EAE.

In MS there is an inverse relationship between involvement of the brain and spinal cord similar to that in chronic relapsing EAE. This is best exemplified by the cases of spinal MS and Devic's disease where involvement of the brain is minimal, with the exception of the optic nerves. Although involvement of the spinal cord, brain stem, and optic nerves is frequently a feature of acute MS and early relapses of chronic MS, the predominant localization of lesions in these areas is not only due to the severity of the disease in the early chronic phases of MS. There are many examples of rapidly progressive or relapsing MS with short clinical duration with lesions mainly confined to the periventricular white matter.

4.13 The Variability of Inflammatory Demyelinating Lesions

As already discussed individual features of inflammatory demyelinating lesions like demyelination, remyelination, oligodendroglia destruction, sclerosis, etc. vary in intensity in different lesions in MS and chronic relapsing EAE. Each individual aspect is closely interconnected with other lesional features, and, therefore, quantitative changes in a singular aspect may influence the final outcome of a plaque dramatically. Therefore it is not surprising to find a large variety of differently structured chronic lesions in different models or even in different animals within the same model. Many examples of this phenomenon have been already given in earlier chapters and thus only the most characteristic plaques will be discussed here.

The two most common lesions in guinea pigs are: (a) the *demyelinated sclerotic plaque* (Fig. 21), which is sharply demarcated from the surrounding white matter and characterized by demyelination, oligodendroglia loss, pronounced sclerosis, and poor remyelination and (b) the *partially or completely remyelinated plaque* with moderate or mild gliosis, relative oligodendroglia preservation, and rapid remyelination (Fig. 19).

Other characteristic lesions are: (c) *the hypercellular plaque* (Figs. 10, 32), mainly found in chronic EAE in rats with numerous stellate microglia-like cells within the lesion and a high proportion of myelin degradation performed in local cells like astrocytes and oligodendrocytes, (d) the *rare destructive lesion* (Fig. 33) with damage to all glial elements including astroglia with relative sparing of axons, and (e) *lesions* with high incidence of *axonal or neuronal destruction.*

Furthermore, all transitional stages of the above-described lesions may be found when a large sample of EAE animals is studied.

In MS the most classical lesion is the demyelinated sclerotic plaque. However, it must be stressed again that in MS too high a variability of the morphology of demyelinated plaques is common. This variability in structural aspects of MS lesions is partly responsible for the large number of sometimes even contradicting pathogenetic interpretations of this disease.

A more detailed study of the development of demyelinated plaques in chronic EAE provides some explanation for this variability at both structural and pathogenetic levels.

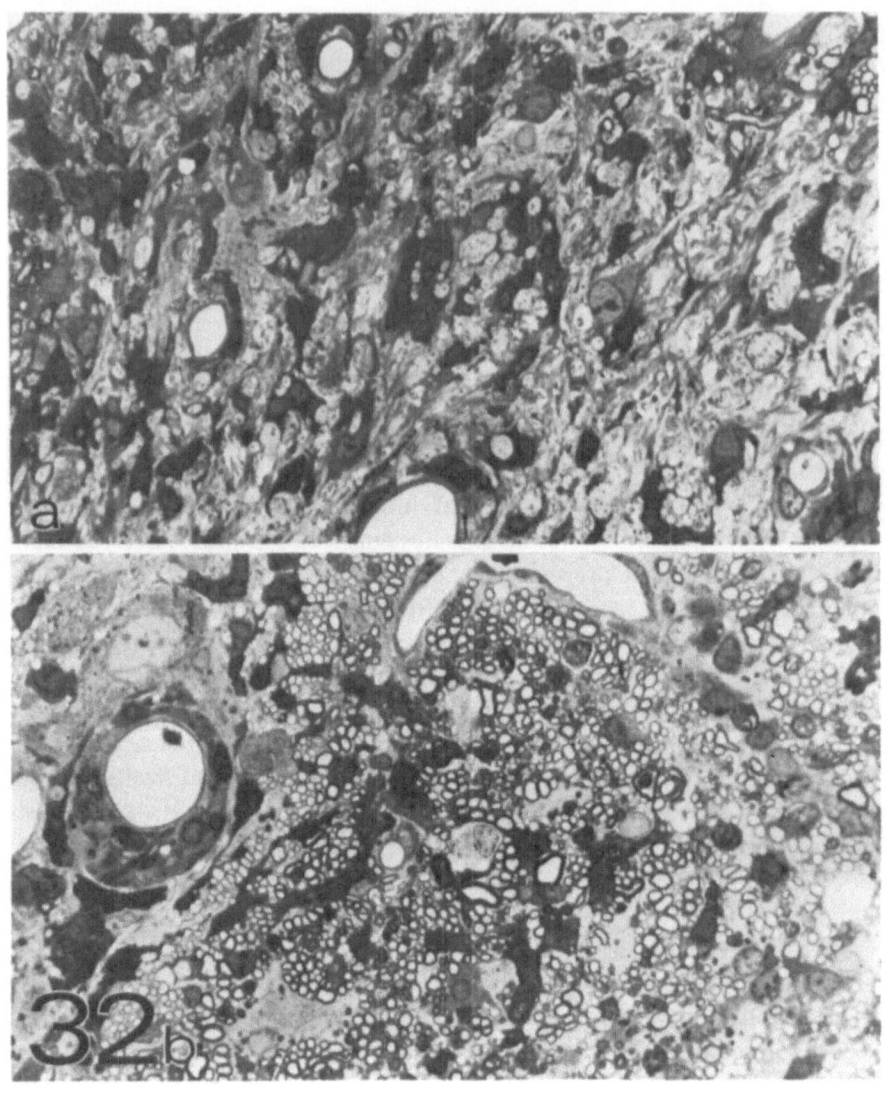

Fig. 32 a, b. Chronic EAE in Sprague Dawley rats. Different stages in the development of demyelinated hypercellular (microglia) lesions. **a** Cerebellar white matter, demyelinated lesion with numerous small, dark, stellate, microglia-like cells. Toluidine blue, x 1000. **b** Dorsal column of the spinal cord; remyelinated lesion; similar microglia-like cells are still present in the lesion. Toluidine blue, x 1000

Fig. 33 a–d. Chronic EAE in Sprague Dawley rats; large destructive lesion in the anterior column of the ▷ spinal cord with ongoing activity and remyelination. **a** Toluidine blue, x 80. **b** Active lesional zone with massive swelling of myelin sheaths and early myelin degradation products. Toluidine blue, x 1000. **c** Inactive, remyelinated zone; the astroglia is completely destroyed, the perivascular and subpial glia limitans is missing, and the nerve fibers are remyelinated by Schwann cells. Toluidine blue, x 1000. **d** Transitional area between active and inactive zone with massive swelling of astrocytes and large protoplasmatic astroglia, containing myelin degradation products. Toluidine blue, x 1000

90

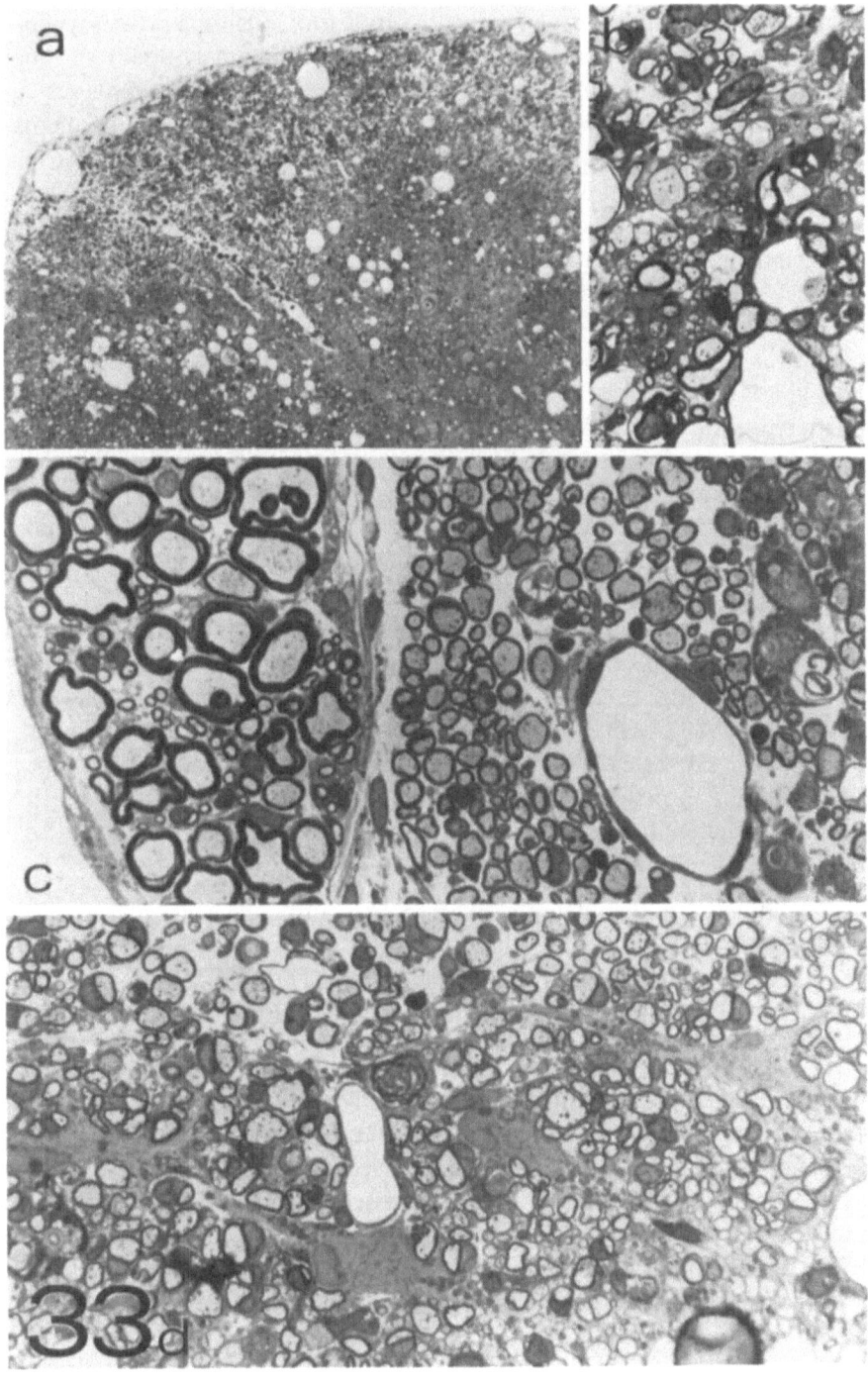

91

The structural interdependency of individual aspects of inflammatory demyelinated lesions has been discussed in detail before and will be only briefly summarized in this chapter. The pattern of demylination (myelin stripping versus vesicular disruption of myelin) as well as the degradation of myelin in local versus hematogenous cells correlates with the number of hematogenous macrophages available in initial perivenous infiltrates. In guinea pigs with a very high number of large mononuclear cells in the lesions, myelin stripping is the dominant mode of demyelination, and myelin degradation is performed mainly in hematogenous cells. This also reflects on vascular and meningeal pathology in this animal model with a high degree of capillary and meningeal fibrosis in chronic lesions. Intense vascular changes, however, will induce pronounced edema which then will also influence the degree of gliosis.

With regarding to central remyelination the extent of destruction of oligodendrocytes in active lesions seems to be an important limiting factor. In addition, the degree of gliosis and other direct factors changing oligodendroglia function (like antibodies against surface antigens) may play a role in preventing remyelination. Peripheral (Schwann cell) remyelination in CNS lesions is augmented when the glia limiting membrane is functionally impaired.

The degree of gliosis is dependent upon the total amount of tissue destruction in the active phase of plaque formation and upon the degree of vascular pathology and edema. Furthermore, glia-stimulating factors produced by inflammatory cells (Fontana et al. 1980a, b) may link the degree of gliosis with the intensity of inflammation in the active stage of demyelination. On the other hand, damage to astrocytes during lesion formation will inhibit subsequent gliosis.

On a pathogenetic level there seem to be mainly four factors governing the final structural outcome of demyelinated lesions:

1. The intensity of the inflammatory response during the active phases of the diseases
2. The time interval between sensitization and plaque formation
3. The degree of compartmentalization of the immune reaction in the CNS
4. The direction of the immune response

It has previously been noted by several investigators that the degree of inflammation during the active stage of EAE largely affects the degree of tissue damage in the lesions, especially also the involvement of secondary targets, like axons, neurons, blood vessels, and others. However, as discussed above, variations in these parameters will also secondarily affect the extent of gliosis and remyelination. The intensity of inflammatory reaction in EAE depends mainly on the sensitization procedure used for the experiments and on the genetic background of the sensitized animal (Alvord 1970; Levine 1974).

The time interval between sensitization and plaque formation plays a role in several features of developing EAE lesions which are best exemplified in the comparison of acute-subacute EAE lesions with chronic plaques. The degree of inflammation decreases; however, the amount of plasma cells in the infilrates increases with time after sensitization. The extent of demyelination, the size of demyelinating lesions, and the destruction of oligodendrocytes increases in newly formed lesions in the chronic stage, whereas the remyelinating capacity decreases. The reason for these time-dependent changes in plaque structure are not yet resolved; there are, however, some immunological parameters in EAE which may serve an explanation for this phenomenon. The delayed hypersensitivity reaction against CNS antigens, especially myelin basic protein, is maximal in intensity in acute EAE as soon as 10 and 20 days after sensitization, whereas the humoral immune response following encephalitogentic challenge in chronic relapsing EAE develops only slowly, reaching maximal levels in this model between 100 and 200 days after sensitization (Mehta et al. 1981; Karcher et al. 1981). In addition, the appearance of antibodies against CNS antigens (MBP, galactocerebroside, and gangliosides) in the sera correlates well with the development of confluent demyelinated plaques in the CNS (Lassmann et al. 1981e). If inflammatory demyelinating lesions may be induced by a cooperation of cellular and humoral immune mechanisms, as suggested by Brosman et al. (1977), Wisniewski et al. (1982), and Lassmann et al. (1981a, d), it is not surprising that changes in their balance will influence the structural expression of the lesions.

The compartmentalization of the immune response in the CNS seems to be mainly responsible for the changes in size, shape, and topographical distribution of the lesions between acute and chronic EAE. Lesions in the acute stage follow a strict perivenous pattern, resulting in relatively even rims of demyelination around the whole venous vascular tree including small postcapillary venoles, medium-sized veins, and large drainage veins. During the chronic stage the lesional morphology changes mainly in three aspects:

The demyelinated lesions, although they may be localized anywhere in the CNS, become more focal than lesions in the acute stage. This results in the formation of large demyelinated plaques, well demarcated from the surrounding, apparently normal white matter.

Some areas of the brain and spinal cord are more frequently involved than others.

The lesions are generally oriented around larger veins or toward the inner and outer surface of the CNS.

The changes in lesional shape and distribution seem to be at least partly due to the seeding of pathogenetically relevant immunocompetent cells in the CNS compartment. Due to anatomical reasons, this seeding of larger amounts of inflammatory cells in the CNS is only possible at certain restricted areas of the CNS parenchyma. It may take place in the loose connective tissue meshwork of the Virchow-Robin spaces which surrounds larger drainage veins, and in the connective tissue of meninges and the choroid plexus. Therefore, following this concept, CNS areas with a high density of drainage veins or others which are covered by meninges should be predilection sites for demyelinated plaques in chronic EAE. This pattern closely resembles that found in the pathohistology of this model (Lassmann et al. 1981a, b). It must be kept in mind, however, that other factors seem to be important for the explanation of lesional topography.

All these above-described factors, although important, cannot fully explain the variability of lesional structure in chronic relapsing EAE – especially the variable degree of damage to oligodendrocytes, astrocytes, and neurons, in addition to the destruction of myelin in lesions with comparable intensity of the inflammatory response. This indicates that in different animals the immune response may be directed against different antigens present not only in myelin but also in astrocytes, oligodendrocytes, and neurons.

4.14 EAE as a Model of Human Inflammatory Demyelinating Diseases

The detailed comparison of the clinical and pathohistological features of EAE with those in human inflammatory demyelinating diseases shows the close similarity of both disease entities. From the view point of pathology it seems especially important that not only the essential structural aspects of inflammatory demyelinating lesions (i.e., inflammation, demyelination, and sclerosis) are mimiced but that in addition the whole variable spectrum of pathohistological changes of these diseases is covered by the model.

In spite of the similarities it must be stressed that there are several aspects which are different in the human disease and the experimental model.

1. The Size of the Demyelinated Lesions. It is evident that lesions in the CNS of small rodents have to be smaller than those in primates and humans. However, the small size of the lesions has several consequences on the pathohistological expression of the lesions. As an example, radial plaque growth is a relatively rare mechanism of lesion enlargement in EAE. In human as well as in experimental demyelinating lesions radial plaque growth is found only in plaques larger than one to several millimeters in diameters. Smaller lesions are demyelinated more synchronously, characterized by the presence of myelin degradation products scattered in the whole lesion. In guinea pigs, however, due to anatomical reasons, lesions of several millimeters in diameter are found only in selected areas of the CNS, especially in the spinal cord. Even in these lesions further enlargement of the plaques is restricted, due to the small size of the tissue. Furthermore, the active zone in radially expanding MS lesions in general is larger than the whole plaques in guinea pigs. Thus radial plaque growth, although present in EAE, is rather an exceptional mechanism of lesion enlargement.

Remyelination is another example of how plaque size influences the structural expression of the lesions. When the borders of inactive chronic MS lesions are studied in detail, generally a zone of reduced myelin density of 0.5 to several millimeters is found. This zone represents an area of remyelination in the majority of

94

cases. When, however, as in EAE in guinea pigs, the diameter of demyelinated plaques is not larger than 1–3 millimeters, complete remyelination of the whole plaque will eventually develop. This may also be one of the reasons for the more effective remyelination in the small lesions of acute MS than in typical chronic MS plaques.

2. The Duration of the Disease. Typical chronic MS is a disease with a duration of several years. On the contrary in chronic EAE even in the most chronic models active disease has not been observed later than 12–15 months after sensitization. As has been discussed in detail, disease duration in EAE affects several pathohistological aspects of demyelinating lesions, including the intensity of inflammation, the extent of oligodendroglia destruction, remyelination, and sclerosis. In the late stage of chronic relapsing EAE, lesions are found which are comparable to typical chronic MS plaques. They are, however, relatively infrequent in comparison with early chronic lesions which mimic the plaques found in acute MS. The reason for this observation is that in the majority of chronic EAE animals the disease is more severe in the early chronic than in the late chronic stage of the disease. The differences in disease duration cannot be explained simply by the different life span of small rodents and humans as even in primates and in allergic encephalomyelitis in humans a longer disease course has not been observed.

3. The Induction of the Disease. Experimental allergic encephalomyelitis is induced by active sensitization of susceptible animals with CNS antigens and adjuvants. Although it is at present unresolved what mechanisms are responsible for keeping the disease active in the chronic stage, some observations suggest that also the duration of the chronic disease is related to the persistence of sensitizing material at the inoculation site (Wisniewski et al. 1982). This observation may to some extent explain the comparatively short disease duration in chronic EAE. In human inflammatory demyelinating diseases it is not known what factors are responsible for disease induction and for the persistence of a chronic or chronic relapsing disease course.

The active immunization in EAE, however, reflects on several immunological parameters in this model. As an example the humoral immune response in the circulation of EAE animals is much more pronounced than in human inflammatory demyelinating diseases (Karcher et al., 1982; Karcher et al. in preparation). A similar elevated humoral immune response in the serum is also observed in animals, sensitized with complete Freund's adjuvant alone, in animals which never develop neurological disease (Karcher et al., in preparation). Therefore using experimental allergic encephalomyelitis as a model of human inflammatory demyelinating diseases, it must always be kept in mind that the etiology of these two diseases may be different. However, the close similarity of clinical and pathohistological aspects of the diseases suggests that EAE is a suitable model for the study of pathogenetic factors involved in the formation of the lesions.

5 Immunopathogenetic Considerations

Although there are evident differences in the etiology, induction, and probably also maintenance between EAE and human inflammatory demyelinating diseases, there is a striking similarity between both conditions regarding the structural features and the evolution of the lesions in the central nervous system. These similarities make possible the conclusion that immunopathological mechanisms play a key role in the pathogenesis of human inflammatory demyelinating diseases. Thus our knowledge of the pathogenetic mechanisms involved in the animal model may be relevant for the understanding of the human diseases. There is a large number of original studies and reviews dealing with this topic available (Frick 1979; Lisak 1980; Wisniewski et al. 1982). For this reason only a few aspects will be discussed in the following chapters; these seem to be the most relevant for an understanding of the pathohistology of inflammatory demyelinating lesions.

5.1 Transfer Studies

When transfer studies are discussed in human diseases, the main interest is focused upon the induction of the disease in normal recipient animals with a transmissable agent. Several reports have claimed the isolation of virus from MS patients including herpes (Gudnadottir et al. 1964), parainfluenza virus (Ter Meulen et al. 1972; Field et al. 1972), "multiple sclerosis associated agent" (Carp et al. 1972), measles (Pertschuk et al. 1976), "bone marrow agent" (Mitchell et al. 1979), cytomegalovirus (chimpanzee agent; Rorke et al. 1979), and corona virus (Burks et al. 1979). In all these instances reproduction in other laboratories has either failed or has not yet been performed. In addition it is not clear to what extent laboratory contaminations play a role in these studies (Sever and Madden 1980). With the "chimpanzee agent" (Rorke et al. 1979) a demyelinating disease was induced after inoculation in monkeys. As, however, the inoculated material contained brain tissue, it cannot be excluded that some kind of experimental allergic encephalomyelitis was induced.

A different approach in transfer studies is the induction of the disease or of elements of the disease immunologically by the use of serum factors or living lymph node cells in vitro and in vivo. Many studies have been performed in this respect which give valuable information regarding the pathogenesis of inflammatory demyelinating lesions in EAE and MS.

1. Serum-Induced Demyelination In Vitro in EAE. When organotypic myelinated CNS tissue cultures are exposed to sera from animals suffering from experimental allergic encephalomyelitis induced by whole CNS tissue, white matter, or myelin, selective demyelination of the myelinated nerve fibers can be observed in the cultures (Bornstein and Appel 1961). Furthermore, such sera may also inhibit myelination in cultures, when applied just prior to or during the period of myelination (Bornstein and Raine 1970; Seil et al. 1975). Demyelination is a selective process; nerve cells and their processes are generally unaffected (Raine and Bornstein 1970a). Oligodendrocytes are also destroyed, provided the cultures are exposed for sufficient time to the demyelinating sera (Raine and Bornstein 1970a). Furthermore, some reactive proliferation of astrocytes may be observed together with increase in size and fibrillar content (Raine and Bornstein 1970b).

Immunologically this in vitro demyelinating activity of EAE sera is confined to the immunoglobulin fraction, due to antibodies from the IgG as well as IgM class (Grundke-Iqbal et al. 1981). The reaction is complement dependent (Appel and Bornstein 1964). Inactivation of complement by heating the sera or by preincubation with zymosan abolishes the demyelinating activity. The activity, however, can be restored by addition of fresh serum as a source of complement (Grundke-Iqbal et al. 1981). The immunoglobulin complement interaction seems to be species specific (Grundke-Iqbal et al. 1981).

Decomplemented EAE sera do not induce demyelination in cultures, but produce profound changes of oligodendroglia structure and behavior together with marked swelling of myelin sheaths (Raine et al. 1978c; Grundke-Iqbal et al. 1981).

2. In Vivo Effect of EAE Sera on Myelin. Considering the demyelinating activity of EAE sera in vitro, several attempts have been made to induce a similar effect in vivo. However, injection of EAE sera into the circulation of normal recipient animals were ineffective (Paterson 1971). This result can be explained by the existence of a blood-brain barrier which allows only a low proportion of immunoglobulins to enter the brain under normal conditions (Tourtellotte et al. 1980). Furthermore, sera will be diluted after injection in the circulation, and concentrations similar to those in in vitro conditions are therefore difficult to obtain.

Jankovic et al. (1965) and Simon and Simon (1975) injected EAE sera into the cerebrospinal fluid of normal recipient animals and described the occurrence of inflammation and demyelination in the CNS of recipient animals. Similar observations were made by Williams et al. (1980) after injection of EAE sera directly into the white matter. Demyelination in all these studies, however, has not been convincingly demonstrated. Saida et al. (1978b, 1979c) observed that sera from EAE and EAN animals as well as sera from animals sensitized with galactocerebrosides may induce demyelination in normal animals when injected into the sciatic nerve. Similarly to in in vitro experiments, demylination was only induced with sera which contained complement. The role of macrophages in the pathogenesis of the lesions was not elucidated.

Since all the above-mentioned studies were carried out with sera from animals with acute EAE, we recently reinvestigated the question of serum-induced demyelination in vivo using sera from different stages of chronic relapsing EAE. In this study undiluted sera from chronic EAE and control animals were injected in the lumbosacral spinal subarachnoid space of normal recipient rats, and the spinal cord and roots were investigated 48 h later for demyelination in the central and peripheral nervous system (Lassmann et al. 1981c).

Sera from animals which were sampled during the acute stage of chronic relapsing EAE showed no or only minimal demyelinating activity, and no demyelination was found with control sera. On the contrary the majority of sera from animals sampled during the chronic stage of the disease were able to induce demyelination in the central as well as peripheral nervous system of normal recipient animals. Thus as a general pattern the appearance of demyelinating activity in the sera correlates with the appearance of large demyelinated plaques in the CNS of the donor animals. However, a clear-cut correlation between serum-demyelinating activity and extent of demyelination in individual donor animals was not present. This was especially the case in animals sampled during the late chronic stage of the disease, where sera sometimes did not show demyelinating activity in spite of ongoing active demyelination in the CNS. Also some strongly demyelinating sera were obtained from animals with completely inactive disease in the CNS. This discrepancy may be best explained by the fact that the blood-brain barrier is partially repaired in the late chronic stage of the disease, and thus parameters measured in the serum do not necessarily reflect the events in the CNS.

The ultrastructural features of demyelination observed in recipient animals following injection of EAE sera into the CSF were similar to those observed in the CNS and PNS of the donor animals. Most frequently vesicular disruption of myelin and to a smaller degree myelin stripping was observed. The extent of demyelination in the central versus the peripheral nervous system varied, some sera predominantly demyelinating peripheral and others central myelin or both. There was a statistically significant relationship between the demyelinating activity of chronic EAE sera and the presence of antibodies directed against CNS antigens (Lassmann et al. 1981e).

The mechanisms leading to demyelination in recipient animals following injection of EAE sera into the cerebrospinal fluid have not yet been completely resolved. When sera from guinea pigs with chronic EAE were injected into the CSF of rats (heterologous system), guinea pig complement was required. Decomplementation by heat inactivation or with zymosan abolished the demyelinating activity. Activity was restored by addition of fresh guinea pig serum to the inactivated EAE serum as a source of complement. On the contrary in a homologous system when sera from rats with chronic EAE were injected into rats, complement inactivation had no effect on the demyelinating activity. Since also no complement was

98

detectable in the CSF of the recipient animals after injection of EAE or control sera, complement seems to play no role in the induction of demyelination in the homologous system (Lassmann et al. 1983). Although definite evidence is not yet available, demyelination in the homologous system may be induced in an interaction between antibodies and activated macrophages similar to that described by Brosnan et al. (1977) as "antibody dependent cell mediated" demyelination.

3. Induction of Demyelination In Vitro with Lymph Node Cells or Peripheral Blood Lymphocytes. Arnason et al. (1969) described demyelination in peripheral nerve cultures following exposure to cells obtained from lymph nodes or peripheral blood derived from animals sensitized for experimental allergic neuritis. Demyelinating activity was found by cells from donor animals sampled as early as 4 days after sensitization; the maximum demyelinating activity was observed when donor animals were sampled between 6 and 9 days after sensitization. In contrast, sera from the same donor animals showed much less demyelinating activity, and the highest titers of demyelinating activity in the sera were found later in the course of the disease (13–15 days after sensitization). There are, however, several doubts regarding the interpretation of these findings. Not only cells from animals sensitized with PNS antigens but also from some of the animals sensitized with kidney homogenate were able to demyelinate the cultures. Furthermore, the demyelinating activity was blocked when anti-IgA was added to the cultures. Thus antibodies seem to play a role in demyelination also in this system.

Bornstein and Iwanami (1971) were able to show that lymph node cells from animals sensitized with CNS antigens were capable of demyelinating nerve fibers in vitro; demyelination, however, was restricted to central myelin. In contrast to the results described by Arnason et al. (1969), sera from EAE animals when supplied with a sufficient amount of complement showed a higher demyelinating activity than lymph node cells. Furthermore, lymph node cells cultured in isolation secreted demyelinating factors into the nutrient medium.

Yonezawa et al. (1980), by studying the morphological changes in cultures in more detail, emphasized another problem in interpretation of the results. These authors differentiated between two tissue alterations induced by the presence of lymph node cells from EAE and EAN animals in the cultures:

Cytotoxic alterations were found most frequently and affected not only myelin sheaths but also all other tissue elements (axons, nerve cells, and glia).

The other alteration, the "activated phagocytosis," was specifically directed against myelin sheaths; it was less frequently observed and did not require complement. However, direct contact of applied lymph node cells to myelin was not clearly demonstrated, and specific myelin destruction was found only when lymph node cells were kept in the cultures for more than 2 days. When cultures were exposed to purified lymphokines mainly cytotoxic changes were observed instead of selective demyelination.

Therefore, none of these experiments provide definitive evidence that sensitized lymphocytes are able to induce selective demyelination in vitro in the absence of antibodies. Furthermore, it must be kept in mind that isolated lymph node cells contain T- as well as B-lymphocytes and thus may contain a proportion of cells producing demyelinating antibodies.

4. In Vitro Passive Transfer of Acute EAE by Means of Lymphocytes. Experimental allergic encephalomyelitis was first successfully transferred in parabiosis experiments (Lipton and Freund 1953). It is now well established that this transfer is induced by sensitized lymphocytes (Paterson 1960; Aström and Waksman 1962). The intensity of transferred disease is directly related to the number of transferred lymphocytes and to their ability to survive in the host environment (Paterson 1960; Aström and Waksman 1962). Furthermore the severity of the disease in recipient animals can be further augmented by selecting the optimal stage of the disease in donor animals and by the mode of transfer. When the blood-brain barrier in recipient animals is circumvented by either injection of lymphocytes into the CSF or by damaging the brain prior to transfer, lesions develop earlier and are generally more severe than after injection of comparable numbers of cells into the circulation of normal animals (Aström and Waksman 1962; Levine 1974).

Passive transfer of lymph node cells from EAE animals generally leads to a mild or clinically silent inflammatory disease of the central nervous system 1–8 days after transfer. In pathohistology perivenous inflammation in the meninges and in the CNS parenchyma is the dominant feature. When higher numbers of sensitized cells are injected directly into the CSF, larger lesions may be induced, characterized by total tissue necrosis with dominant Wallerian type of nerve fiber destruction (Aström and Waksman 1962). Selective demyelination, if observed at all, is restricted to a few nerve fibers adjacent to inflammatory cuffs or in the edge zones of necrotic lesions. Thus the pathology is in contrast to the typical picture of subacute or chronic EAE, where demyelination is the leading aspect of the pathology.

Induction of a chronic demyelinating type of EAE by passive transfer of lymphocytes has so far not been achieved. Injection of sensitized lymphocytes into newborn guinea pigs results in a similar clinical and pathohistological disease pattern to that described above and does not induce a chronic disease (Stone et al. 1968). Passive transfer studies using animals with chronic relapsing EAE as lymphocyte donors have not been successful.

5. In Vitro and In Vivo Studies in Multiple Sclerosis. Compared with EAE, a similar demyelinating activity of patients' sera has been observed in multiple sclerosis in vitro (Bornstein and Appel 1965). The intensity of the demyelinating activity of MS sera correlated well with the clinical course of the disease. The more severe the clinical course the higher the demyelinating activity of sera observed (Lumsden 1971). Furthermore, the demyelinating activity of sera seemed to increase at the beginning of an exacerbation of the disease and decrease during the remission (Lumsden 1971).

The interpretation of these findings, however, is more difficult than interpretation of those obtained in EAE, for several reasons:

Not all but only about 80% of MS sera show demyelinating activity. Furthermore, there is some demyelinating activity in 18%–25% of sera from patients suffering from neurological diseases other than MS. In addition, even some sera from apparently healthy control patients may demyelinate organotypic cultures (Bornstein and Appel 1965; Hughes and Field 1967; Lumsden 1971). Although the demyelinating activity in control sera is less intense than that found in MS patients, the overlap between demyelinating activity in MS versus control sera casts doubts upon the significance of such a test for the diagnosis of MS.

There seem to be at least two different factors in MS sera which are responsible for demyelination in vitro. One factor appears to be immunoglobulin which induces demyelination via activation of the complement system (Grundke-Iqbal and Bornstein 1980). This factor is mainly present in patients with acute exacerbations of the disease (Dowling et al. 1968; Lumsden 1971; Grundke-Iqbal and Bornstein 1980). The other factor is less well defined. It is a heat-labile factor, possibly a proteolytic enzyme (Grundke-Iqbal and Bornstein 1980).

In summary, there seem to be two main differences between in vitro demyelinating activity of EAE versus MS sera:
1. The presence of an unspecific demyelinating factor in human sera (not only in MS sera but also in some obtained from patients with other neurological diseases or control patients). This factor may mask the specific demyelinating activity of immunoglobulins directed against myelin components.
2. The lack of a specific immunoglobulin and complement-related demyelinating activity of sera from MS patients with inactive or with typical mild exacerbating and remitting chronic disease. This latter point, however, does not seem to be a real difference between EAE and MS. Also in chronic relapsing EAE the incidence of in vivo demyelinating activity of sera decreases with the chronicity of the disease. Thus, also sera from animals with late chronic EAE may show only mild or absent demyelinating activity in spite of active demyelination in the CNS. This phenomenon may be due to partial repair of the blood-brain barrier and compartmentalization of the immune reaction in the brain.

Only a few studies are available concerning the transfer of demyelination by lymphocytes in multiple sclerosis and its peripheral counterpart idiopathic polyneuritis Guillian-Barré. Whereas Arnason et al. (1969) were not able to induce demyelination in peripheral nerve cultures with lymphocytes derived from patients with polyneuritis, Yonezawa et al. (1980) found qualitatively similar changes in cultures exposed to cells derived from experimental animals and patients. Also Lumsden (1971) described transfer of demyelination in organotypic cultures with the use of lymphocytes derived from MS patients. However, in all these studies the same difficulties in interpretation as already discussed for EAE are valid.

In spite of the large number of studies dealing with the induction of demyelination in vitro, there are only sporadic reports of comparable studies in vivo. Injection of MS sera into the rat sciatic nerve did not induce demyelination of peripheral nerve fibers (Silberberg et al. 1980). On the contrary, sera from patients with the Guillain-Barré syndrome were able to induce demyelination in a similar in vivo assay (Feasby et al. 1980; Cook and Dowling 1981). However, some demyelination was noted also with control sera (Cook and Dowling 1981). Moreover other experiments with intraneural injections of Guillain-Barré sera did not confirm these studies (Server et al. 1979; Tandon et al. 1980). Therefore, further in vivo studies must be performed with sera from different stages of inflammatory polyradiculitis and MS and by using central myelin as target.

6. Transfer Studies with Cerebrospinal Fluid of EAE Animals and MS Patients. Both EAE and MS are diseases which primarily affect the central nervous system. As already discussed, the immune reaction in both diseases is at least partially compartmentalized in the CNS. Furthermore, the presence of immunoglobulin-containing plasma cells and intrathecal immunoglobulin synthesis has been observed (Grundke-Iqbal et al. 1980; Tourtellotte 1970; Esiri 1977; Mehta et al. 1981). It is surprising at first that only a few data are available about in vitro and in vivo demyelinating activity of cerebrospinal fluid in these diseases. In EAE this may be explained by the extremely small volumes of CSF which can be obtained from small rodents. In MS, demyelinating activity was shown in vitro when concentrated CSF or brain extracts were tested (Lamoureaux and Borduas 1966; Hughes and Field 1967; Kim et al. 1970; Lumsden 1971). Furthermore, there was a good correlation between demyelinating activity and IgG content of the CSF and brain extracts (Kim et al. 1970). In a more recent study, Tabira et al. (1976) showed myelinotoxicity of unconcentrated MS-CSF in the tadpole optic nerve in vivo, which, however, did not lead to complete demyelination. Thus it appears that demyelinating activity of CSF is lower than that found in the serum of the same patients. As there is only a limited barrier between the CSF and the CNS tissue, antibodies directed against surface antigens of CNS components will be partially or totally removed by the excess of antigen. Thus the majority of immunoglobulin detectable in the CSF is probably not directed against CNS antigens and may represent an epiphenomenon of the disease unrelated to the pathogenesis of the lesions.

5.2 The Possible Role of Autoantigens in the Pathogenesis of Inflammatory Demyelinating Lesions

Cellular and humoral immune reactions against a variety of CNS antigens have been described in EAE as well as in MS. These studies have been summarized in detail in recent reviews (Caspary 1977; Frick 1979; Alvord et al. 1979; Arnon et al. 1980; Lisak 1980). Even in EAE there is, however, only fragmentary evidence available on to what extent these immune reactions are actively involved in the pathogenesis of the disease or are secondary to demyelination and liberation of antigen.

In EAE it is now well established that myelin basic protein is the main or even the sole antigen responsible for the induction of the disease (Kies et al. 1960; Roboz Einstein et al. 1962). Proteolipid which as been claimed to be encephalitogenic (Waksman 1959) has been found ineffective when highly purified fractions (Agrawal et al. 1977) were used. More recently an encephalitogenic fraction of myelin has been described (Lipophilin, Hashim et al. 1980), which, however, showed some cross reactivity with myelin basic protein.

Although myelin basic protein may induce a perivenous leukoencephalitis in experimental animals, it alone does not seem to be an effective antigen for induction of widespread demyelination. In acute EAE induced by MBP, Lampert and Kies (1967) showed demyelination in the vicinity of vessels with inflammatory cuffs. However, a similar pattern and extent of myelin destruction may also be found as an unspecific consequence of delayed hypersensitivity reactions in the CNS directed against antigens, unrelated to myelin (Wisniewski and Bloom 1975). Induction of chronic EAE with MBP is difficult (Wisniewski et al. 1980a, 1982). Panitch and Ciccone (1981) described a chronic relapsing form of EAE in rats following sensitization with MBP. Pathohistology in these animals, however, revealed chronic leukoencephalitis without the presence of plaque-like demyelination. Similar observations have also been made in our own experiments in guinea pigs. On the other hand, Alvord (1980) described the occurrence of large demyelinated plaques in monkeys, induced by repeated sensitization with MBP. However, the extremely low incidence of this finding raises the possibility that other factors than MBP were involved in the induction of the lesions. Also Colover (1980) observed large demyelinated lesions after MBP sensitization. In these experiments, however, presensitization of the animals with ovalbumin and a synthetic adjuvant was necessary. The exact role of these two additional antigens in the pathogenesis of the lesions is still unresolved.

Thus, as far as it is known so far, CNS antigens other than MBP do not seem able to induce an autoimmune encephalitis. This is different from observations in the peripheral nervous system. A demyelinating polyradiculoneuritis may be induced by hyperimmunization with galactocerebrosides (Saida et al. 1979b) and gangliosides (Nagai et al. 1976). This difference of susceptibility between the central and pripheral nervous system seems to be due to the presence of the blood-brain barrier, which is more effective than the blood-nerve barrier (Waksman 1960a).

There are some indications that antigens other than MBP may play an additional role in the pathogenesis of inflammatory demyelinating lesions. As already discussed, sera from EAE animals may induce demyelination in vitro and also in vivo following injection into peripheral nerves or into the cerebrospinal fluid of normal recipient animals. As determined in in vitro experiments, antigens responsible for the induction of demyelinating antibodies have been found to be galactocerebroside (Dubois-Dalqu et al. 1970; Saida et al. 1979b) or other chemically less well-defined antigens from myelin (Lebar et al. 1976, 1979) or oligodendroglia (Saida et al. 1977). MBP, myelin-associated glycoprotein, and proteolipid protein have been shown to be ineffective (Seil et al. 1968, 1981; Seil and Agrawal 1980). Similarly in in vivo models demyelination has been induced by antigalactocerebroside sera (Saida et al. 1979a).

Recently we have been able to induce demyelination in normal recipient animals by injection of antiganglioside serum into the cerebrospinal fluid (Lassmann et al. 1981e). In addition to demyelination, profound alterations of blood vessel walls and astroglia were observed after application of antiganglioside sera.

All these in vitro and in vivo experiments indicate that antibodies directed against surface antigens of the myelin sheath may induce damage to the nervous system, provided they are able to penetrate the blood-brain barrier or are produced locally in the CNS compartment and a proper effector mechanism is available.

There are at present few studies available showing a modification of MBP-induced EAE by the presence of additional CNS antigens in the inoculation material. In acute EAE the clinical course and the pathohistological alterations may be modified when glactocerebrosides or acidic brain proteins are used for sensitization in addition to MBP (Brostoff and Powers 1975; Yasuda et al. 1975). Nagai et al. (1980) have shown that the purely inflammatory type of experimental allergic neuritis induced by P_2 protein may be converted into a demyelinating type of EAN, similar to that found after sensitization with whole peripheral nerve, when gangliosides are added to the sensitization medium. Similarly a chronic demyelinating type of EAE, although with low incidence, is noted when animals are sensitized with MBP together with myelin lipids or with a crude protein fraction of myelin (Madrid et al. 1981a). It must be noted, however, that the incidence of chronic demyelinating EAE and the extent of demyelination in individual animals in these experiments was much lower than is generally found after sensitization with whole spinal cord tissue.

The direct determination of antigens responsible for induction of inflammatory demyelinating lesions in EAE is complicated by the fact that any interference with the integrity of native spinal cord prior to sensitization apparently reduces the incidence and severity of the chronic demyelinating disease (Schwerer et al. 1981a). Even when myelin instead of native spinal cord is used for sensitization, the incidence of chronic demyelinating EAE is lower and the size of individual demyelinated lesions is small (Madrid et al. 1981a).

5.3 Conclusions

5.3.1 The Variability of EAE Lesions as an Expression of Multiple Antigens and Effector Mechanisms

It is now well established that the perivenous leukoencephalomyelitis of acute EAE is induced by a cellular immune response and that myelin basic protein is the most relevant if not even the only antigen responsible (Waksman and Morrison 1951; Paterson 1960; Kies et al. 1960; Roboz Einstein et al. 1962; Bernard 1976; Ortiz-Ortiz and Weigle 1976). Similarly, chronic EAE is induced only when MBP is present in the sensitization medium (Schwerer et al. 1981a; Madrid et al. 1981a). There is at present not much evidence available on what immunological mechanisms are reponsible for the chronic course of the disease, although some experiments suggest that the onset of an exacerbation correlates with fluctuations of T-cell subpopulations (Traugott et al. 1979). There are several indications that other (additional?) mechanisms may play a role in the expression of a chronic demyelinating type of EAE.

Passive transfer studies with lymp node cells have not yet resulted in the induction of a chronic demyelinating type of EAE. Induction of demyelination in vitro with lymph node cells has not been convincingly demonstrated, since in the positive reports either no clear distinction between selective demyelination and cytotoxicity was made or the role of antibodies in the pathogenesis of demyelination was not excluded. More recently selective destruction of oligodendrocytes in vitro was described by a cellular immune response against galactocerebroside (Niedieck and Lohmann 1981), although in this experimental system it is also not clear whether a direct cellular-cytotoxicity- or an antibody-dependent cellular cytotoxicity is responsible for the damage. Injection of lymph node cells from EAE animals into the CNS compartment in vivo induced unspecific tissue damage rather than selective demyelination (Aström and Waksman 1962).

In the model of chronic relapsing EAE there is a striking difference between the pathology of the lesions in the active disease in the acute stage and the pathology of those in the chronic stage. Whereas acute EAE is a predominantly inflammatory disease with little or no demyelination, widespread plaque-like demyelination is the leading event in the pathology of chronic EAE. There are several possible explanations for this phenomenon.

There may be differences in the intensity and duration of inflammation between acute and chronic EAE. This explanation, however, seems to be unlikely, as the intensity of inflammation in acute EAE is generally higher than that found in the chronic stage of the disease. Furthermore, persistence of inflammation and clinically active disease in the acute-subacute stage of chronic relapsing EAE for 2 or 3 weeks does not lead to plaque-like demyelination of the lesions. On the contrary, large confluent demyelinated plaques in chronic relapsing EAE may develop within 2–3 days of onset of a relapse.

Another possible explanation for the differences in the pathology of acute and chronic EAE is that the cellular composition of inflammatory infiltrates changes. As proteolytic enzymes seem to be involved in the pathogenesis of demyelination (Cammer et al. 1978; Hallpike and Adams 1969; Cuzner and Davison 1979; Smith 1977, 1980), a higher amount of macrophages in the lesions may possibly result in more extensive demyelination. Although there is a relatively high number of phagocytes in chronic EAE lesions at the stage of debris removal, there does not seem to be a striking difference in the cellular composition of the inflammatory infiltrates of initial lesions between acute and chronic EAE, with the exception of high numbers of plasma cells in the latter. Moreover, it is not yet clear by what mechanisms macrophages are activated in EAE lesions and directed against the target structures of myelin.

A third possible explanation for the differences between acute and chronic EAE is that the immune response in the chronic stage is directed against antigens other than in the acute stage of the disease. Humoral and cellular immune responses have been described in EAE or following sensitization of animals with purified CNS components directed against a variety of CNS antigens including ethanolic brain extracts (Paterson et al. 1965), sphingolipids (Yokoyama et al. 1962), galactocerebroside (Niedieck 1975; Schwerer et al. 1981b; Niedieck and Lohmann 1981) and ganglioside (Schwerer et al. 1981b), sulfatide (Schwerer et al. 1981b), M_2 protein of myelin (Lebar et al. 1976, 1979), and oligodendrocytes (Abramsky 1979). However, with the exception of oligodendrocytes, it has so far not been possible to induce an inflammatory demyelinating disease of the CNS by sensitization of susceptible animals with these antigens. The oligodendrocyte fraction contains MBP, which seems to be responsible for EAE induction (McDermott et al. 1977).

A fourth possibility is that in the course of the disease immune response against antigens other than MBP may modify the disease, which is primarily induced by basic protein. There are several observation at least for humoral immune reactions suggesting that they may be involved in the pathogenesis of demyelination. The appearance of large demyelinated plaques in chronic relapsing EAE correlates well with the appearance of a humoral immune response in the sera, CSF, and brain extracts of the animals (Lassmann et al. 1981e). Furthermore, this immune response is at least partly directed against autoantigens of the central nervous system (Schwerer et al. 1981b; Schwerer et al., in preparation) which are responsible for the induction of demyelinating antibodies in vitro and in vivo (Dubois-Dalqc et al. 1970; Saida et al. 1979c; Lassmann et al. 1981e). Furthermore, serum demyelinating activity in vivo in chronic relapsing EAE appears in parallel with the occurrence of plaque-like demyelination in the CNS of donor animals (Lassmann et al 1981c, e). The increased permeability of the blood-brain barrier for immunoglobulins in chronic EAE and the dressing of myelin sheaths with immunoglobulins at the edge of actively demyelinating lesions visualized by immunofluorescence

106

(Grundke-Iqbal et al. 1980) further supports the concept that antibodies are involved in the pathogenesis of demyelination in this model.

It is now well established that EAE cannot be transferred passively by serum injected into the circulation (Paterson 1971). However, the above-mentioned observations indicate that the perivenous inflammatory disease induced by sensitization with MBP may be modified to a massively demyelinating type of disease by the simultaneous presence of antibodies directed against myelin surface antigens.

There are several possible mechanisms by which antibodies directed against myelin or other CNS components may induce damage to the central nervous tissue in EAE. As suggested from the evidence available, demyelination induced by EAE sera in vitro is accomplished by a direct antibody-dependent complement-mediated lysis of the target structures (Appel and Bornstein 1964; Grundke-Iqbal et al. 1981). A similar mechanism may operate in chronic EAE in vivo provided sufficient concentrations of antibodies and complement may reach the CNS tissue through leaking vessels. However, in immunofluorescence studies in chronic relapsing EAE no complement was detected in the lesions in spite of the presence of high amounts of immunoglobulins and active demyelination (Grundke-Iqbal et al. 1980). Furthermore, when EAE sera are injected into the CSF of normal recipient animals, demyelination is induced in the absence of complement provided that the chronic EAE serum and the recipient animal belong to the same species (Lassmann et al., 1983). Although these studies do not exclude that complement may augment the extent of demyelination induced by EAE sera, they clearly indicate that complement is not absolutely required.

Antibodies may also act in the pathogenesis of demyelination in EAE by direct interaction of cellular and humoral immune responses. An interaction between specific antibodies and activated macrophages has been shown to induce demyelination (Brosnan et al. 1977; Wisniewski et al. 1980b) and has been denominated "antibody-dependent cell-mediated demyelination" (Brosnan et al. 1977). Such a direct interaction of humoral and cellular immune mechanisms may be further augmented by the presence of complement (Perlmann et al. 1981). Thus multiple different effector mechanisms may be involved either separately or in cooperation in the destruction of myelin in EAE.

The concept that EAE lesions may be modified by the presence of immune reactions against antigens other than MBP may not only explain the differences in the extent of demyelination between acute and chronic EAE but also the structural variability of chronic EAE lesions. It has been shown in vitro and in vivo that EAE sera or sera from animals sensitized against purified CNS antigens may induce variable damage to individual components of the CNS and PNS. Antisera against galactocerebrosides and M_2 protein mainly affect myelin and the myelin-supporting cells (Dubois-Dalcq et al. 1970; Lebar et al. 1976). However, in chronic EAE in guinea pigs galactocerebroside is not the only antigen responsible for induction of demyelinating antibodies (Lassmann et al. 1981e). Antisera against oligodendrocytes may demyelinate in vitro (Saida et al. 1977) and may bind to oligodendrocytes; this binding is, however, not absorbed by incubation with myelin. Demyelinating activity in CNS and PNS cultures of EAE sera is variable, indicating that different antigens in the CNS and PNS are responsible for the induction of demyelinating activity (Bornstein and Iwanami 1971; Yonezawa et al. 1968). Sera directed against gangliosides may induce damage to myelin, astrocytes, nerve cells, and blood vessels in normal recipient animals in vivo (Karpiak et al. 1976; Schwerer et al., in preparation). In individual chronic EAE animals, antibodies against several different CNS antigens may be found, and the relative proportion of antibodies against CNS antigens varies from animal to animal (Schwerer et al. 1981; Lassmann et al. 1981e). Thus the final pathogenetic event in a single animal may reflect the sum of immune responses against a large variety of antigens. In such a situation a variability in the structural aspects o the lesions must be expected.

5.3.2 The Compartmentalization of the Immune Reaction and Its Consequences for the Study of Chronic EAE Pathogenesis

It is the natural function of the blood-brain barrier to protect the central nervous system from toxic substances which may occur in the circulation (Lee 1971). However, in chronic inflammatory conditions of the CNS a partial or total repair of the blood-brain barrier may entrap inflammatory cells and mediators in the CNS compartment and may thus allow immune reactions in the brain, independent of the regulatory influences of the general immune system (Tourtellotte 1970). In chronic relapsing EAE there are several indications that such compartmentalization of the immune reaction occurs in the CNS. Increased IgG/albumin ratios and oligoclonal IgG bands may be found in brain extracts of affected animals (Mehta et al. 1981). Furthermore, pathohistology in these animals shows the seeding of lymphocytes and plasma cells in the CNS parenchyma and meninges in spite of only low grade or absent blood-brain barrier damage. As has been described in detail earlier this compartmentalization of the immune response has consequences upon the structural expression of the lesions, especially with regard to distribution of inflammatory infiltrates and lesional topography. However, in addition to these aspects of pathohistology immunological parameters will also be influenced by the repaired blood-brain barrier. In such animals data obtained from the serum will no longer reflect the immunological changes occurring in the CNS. As an example during the late chronic phase of chronic relapsing EAE, massive demyelinating activity of the sera of sensitized animals can be found in the absence of active demyelination in the brain and spinal cord of the donor animals and vice versa (Lassmann et al. 1981c).

Therefore, in chronic relapsing EAE the study of pathogenetic factors involved in demyelination must be concentrated on the early chronic phase of the disease. In this stage blood-brain barrier damage is massive, and an exchange of inflammatory cells and mediators between the CNS and the circulation can be anticipated.

Alternatively, studies in the late chronic phase of the disease should focus upon the central nervous system. However, as there is no effective barrier between the CSF and the CNS tissue, autoantibodies in the CSF will be partly or totally absorbed by the excess of antigen. This may explain why no demyelinating activity was found in unconcentrated CSF samples of chronic EAE animals (Lassmann et al., unpublished).

5.3.3 Implications for Future Research in Human Inflammatory Demyelinating Diseases

The possibility that multiple antigens and multiple effector mechanisms play a role in the pathogenesis of inflammatory demyelinating lesions complicates the planning of future studies regarding the pathogenesis in humans. In fact several aspects in multiple sclerosis pathology and immunology indicate that more than a single pathogenetic event or mechanism is responsible for the disease. In this regard it is especially interesting to compare the pathohistology of acute disseminated leukoencephalomyelitis (ADLE) with Marburg's type of acute MS (Marburg 1906). Both diseases show a comparable extent and distribution of perivenous inflammation. However, demyelination is sparse in ADLE and restricted to small perivenous sleeves, whereas in acute MS extensive plaque-like demyelination is the leading event in pathohistology. Transitional stages between ADLE and acute MS can be found, and several authors thus came to the conclusion that these diseases are essentially similar. It must be noted however, that the majority of ADLE cases are arrested in the stage of perivenous demyelination. Furthermore, the extent of demyelination is not merely related to disease duration. In typical ADLE cases demyelination is still restricted to perivenous sleeves, even in cases with a clinical duration of several months. Thus, in analogy to the above-discussed mechanisms in EAE, additional pathogenetic factors seem necessary also in human inflammatory demyelinating diseases to convert the perivenous leukoencephalomyelitis of ADLE into an MS-like disease with large inflammatory demyelinating lesions. It is at present not clear whether chronic MS starts in the first exacerbation with a pathohistological picture of ADLE, although the continuous spectrum of transitional cases of ADLE, acute MS, and chronic MS supports this concept.

Another aspect of pathohistology of MS lesions which indicates that more than one mechanism may be involved in the pathogenesis of the disease is the variability of structural aspects of MS lesions. As has already been discussed, the extent of oligodendroglia loss, remyelination, sclerosis, neuronal and axonal loss, and peripheral nervous system involvement is different from case to case. This variability cannot be explained on the basis of secondary damage due to intensity of the inflammatory reaction or secondary vascular complications alone.

The problems in immunological studies regarding autoimmunity in MS cases are best illustrated by the fact that autosensitization against individual CNS components was never demonstrated in 100% of investigated cases (for review, see Frick 1979). Furthermore, similar tests revealed positive results in a variable proportion of normal controls and patients with other neurological diseases. Results like this, however, must be expected when a combination of different immune mechanisms is required for the induction of the disease and when autosensitization against several different CNS antigens may result in similar tissue damage.

The compartmentalization of the immune response in the CNS is an even more significant problem in MS research than in studies dealing with the pathogenesis of chronic relapsing EAE. In the human disease investigations are mainly performed on cases of chronic MS, in cases where the blood-brain barrier is even less impaired than in the most chronic animals with chronic relapsing EAE. Cases of acute MS which are comparable to the early chronic stage of chronic relapsing EAE would be more appropriate for the study of serum factors and immunocompetent cells in the circulation. These cases, however, are rare and frequently misdiagnosed clinically. As mentioned above studies of autosensitization performed on CSF samples seem to be of limited value because of the lack of an effective barrier between the CNS tissue and the CSF. For this reason for instance autoantibodies in the CSF will be absorbed in the brain and spinal cord by the excess of antigen, and CSF immunoglobulins will mainly contain antibodies directed against antigens, not expressed on the surface of CNS components. This may explain why demyelinating activity in vitro in the CSF of MS patients is found only when the samples are concentrated up to 100-fold (Kim et al. 1970).

The close similarity of the pathology between EAE and MS suggests that similar mechanisms are involved in the pathogenesis of inflammatory demyelinating lesions in humans and in this experimental model.

In recent studies it has been shown that following certain viral infections, demyelinating lesions may be induced in the central nervous system and that autoimmune mechanisms may play a role in the pathogenesis of these lesions (Wisniewski et al. 1972; Krakowka et al. 1973; Koestner et al. 1974; Dal Canto et al. 1979; Steck et al. 1981; Lipton et al. 1980; Dal Canto and Rabinowitz 1982; Watanabe et al. 1982). These studies may represent the link between the etiology of human inflammatory demyelinating diseases and experimental allergic encephalomyelitis. In the light of these studies it seems even more important that in a pure autoimmune model like EAE multiple antigens and effector mechanisms seem to be involved in the disease. Furthermore, it must be emphasized that many autoantigens which may induce immunological damage to the nervous system directly or indirectly are not yet completely characterized chemically, or are even unknown. This aspect at present seems to be the most promising in the study of pathogenesis of inflammatory demyelinating diseases in humans and experimental animals.

6 Addendum: Material and Methods – Models of Chronic EAE

Since the earliest studies dealing with the pathogenesis of multiple sclerosis, it was felt that the existence of a suitable animal model would contribute much to our understanding of this disease. Experimental allergic encephalomyelitis has been regarded as such a model since the first description of a chronic inflammatory demyelinating disease following autosensitization with CNS tissue (Rivers et al. 1933; Ferraro and Cazzullo 1948). In spite of sporadic reports of other chronic extensively demyelinating EAE models more recently, the main research efforts have concentrated on the pathogenesis of acute EAE, a predominantly inflammatory disease with little demyelintion. This surprising development may be explained at least partly by the fact that in general chronic EAE models are difficult to reproduce. Thus in the following chapter a more detailed description of the methods used in the present study will be given, and some of the most important factors which influence the development of chronic demyelinating EAE will be discussed.

6.1 Material and Methods

6.1.1 Animal Care

The present study is based on clinical and pathohistological findings obtained in more than 400 guinea pigs and 42 Sprague Dawley rats, sensitized for chronic relapsing EAE. Guinea pigs included Strain 13 and Hartley strains, obtained from different breeders. Two to five animals were housed together and fed on a commercial compound pelleted diet with water ad libitum. In addition hay or fresh cabbage was supplied to the commercial diet. When fresh cabbage was not available vitamin C was supplemented in the drinking water. Paralyzed animals were given supportive care. The skin was washed and dried daily to prevent pressure sores, and special attention was paid that sick animals were supplied with sufficient food and drinking water.

6.1.2 Clinical Grading

All animals were examined daily for neurological signs. For evaluation of the clinical severity of the disease the following scoring system was used:

Grade 0: well, no signs

Grade 1: weight loss, weakness, decreased activity, no definite neurological disease

Grade 2: Mild paraparesis; animal unsteady on hind limbs, with altered gait or mild spasticity

Grade 3: Moderate paraparesis; highly abnormal gait with hind and front legs splayed apart; incontinence; pronounced spasticity of the extremities

Grade 4: Severe paraplegia or quadriplegia; animal unable to move the involved extremities. Occasionally vestibular signs with abnormal posture

Grade 5: Moribund, convulsions, impaired respiration

Although this grading system proved to be valuable in the clinical exploration of diseased animals, it must be kept in mind that mainly spinal cord and brain stem lesions are recorded. Animals with exclusive involvement of the periventricular white matter, even with very large lesions, are frequently graded grade 0 or 1 in this scoring system. Furthermore, the clinical status in animals with inactive lesions in the CNS may deteriorate during secondary complications in the colony, like infectious diseases. Thus a relapse of the disease may be simulated in the absence of active lesions in the nervous system. In addition, it must be considered that it is nearly impossible in small rodents to differentiate between CNS or PNS disease on clinical evaluation alone.

6.1.3 Sensitization Procedure

The inoculation medium was prepared according to the method described by Wisniewski and Keith (1977). One gram Hartley guinea pig spinal cord was homogenized in 1 ml saline and 2 ml Difco Complete Adjuvant (Difco H37Ra) in a Sorvall Omnimixer. Before homogenization 10 mg/ml heat-inactivated mycobacterium (Difco H37Ra) was added to the inoculum. The emulsion was always prepared fresh immediately before sensitization. As will be discussed below, various amounts of this emulsion were applied into the dorsum of the hind legs or in addition into the nuchal area. The age of the animals at the time of sensitization was variable. In guinea pigs animals were sensitized either newborn or during the juvenile period (3-35 days after birth). Sprague Dawley rats were sensitized between the age of 1 week and 4 months.

6.1.4 Sampling of Animals

Animals were sampled depending upon the clinical course of the disease. Special care was taken to investigate all stages of the disease by sequential sampling of animals with comparable clinical disease. Following exsanguination and cerebrospinal fluid puncture the animals were generally perfused via the aorta. The following fixatives were used for perfusion: 4% phosphate buffered paraformaldehyde, a mixture of 0.5% paraformaldehyde and 1.5% glutaraldehyde, 3% glutaraldehyde, or Müller's fixation solution for impregnation of degenerating myelin (Marchi reaction). For frozen sections animals were perfused with buffered saline (Grundke-Iqbal et al. 1980). Animals which died unexpextedly during the experiments were dissected and the tissue samples immersed in 10% buffered formalin solution.

After perfusion a general autopsy was performed in the animals, and the following tissue samples embedded for light and electron microscopy: brain, spinal cord, including the meninges and roots, trigeminal root, sciatic nerve, brachial plexus and the sensitization site. In addition, other organs which macroscopically appeared abnormal were embedded for light microscopy. As during the experiments it became evident that a large number of investigated tissue blocks are a prerequisite for accurate information about pathohistology in EAE, the entire brain and spinal cord were embedded for light and electron microscopy. The evaluation of PNS pathology in chronic EAE was mainly focused upon the spinal and cranial roots, because the highest number of lesions was found in this location.

Light microscopic stains included hematoxylin eosin, luxol fast blue, cresyl violet, Bodian, Sudan III, Sudan black B, periodic acid Schiff reaction, Marchi reaction, phosphotungstic acid hematoxylin, Holzer's glia stain, Prussian blue, and Weil-Davenports silver impregnation for oligodendroglia and microglia. For electron microscopy glutaraldehyde-fixed tissue samples were postfixed in osmic acid and routinely embedded in Epon.

Meningeal pathology was studied on isolated stretch preparations of the pia mater (Kitz et al. 1981). Leptomeninges were stained with toluidine blue, Sudan black B-nuclear fast red, or osmicated and embedded for electron microscopy.

Blood-brain barrier-studies were performed either with immunofluorescence for serum proteins (Grundke-Iqbal et al. 1980) or in animals injected with horseradish peroxidase (Boehringer grade II) 1 h before sampling. To avoid anaphylactic reaction due to HRP injection the animals were pretreated with Benadryl (2 mg/kg). These animals were perfused with the above-described formaldehyde-glutaraldehyde mixture and small tissue slices or frozen sections incubated in diaminobenzidine medium according to the method described by Reese and Karnovsky (1967). Following histochemical visualization of HRP-reaction product, samples were either directly studied light microscopically or immersed in osmic acid, embedded in Epon, and studied with the electron microscope.

6.1.5 Human Material

Studies on multiple sclerosis pathology were performed on the material collected in the Neurological Institute during the past decades. A more detailed light microscopic survey of this material has previously been given by Jellinger (1969) and Guseo and Jellinger (1975). For the present study special cases were selected according to the clinical course and light microscopic pathology. They included cases of acute MS according to the definition of Marburg (1906), cases of chronic MS with recent exacerbations and histochemically active lesions in the CNS, and cases with extensive shadow plaque formation. Human material was fixed in 10% neutral formalin solution. Light microscopy was performed on frozen and paraffin sections with the same staining methods as described above. Following light microscopic examination, tissue blocks corresponding to selected light microscopically intersting areas were dissected out, postfixed in osmic acid, and embedded for electron microsopy.

6.2 Factors Modifying the Development of Chronic EAE Models

6.2.1 Guinea Pig Strains

Similarly to in acute EAE the genetic background of the sensitized animals plays an important role in the induction of chronic EAE (Stone et al. 1969). Whereas Strain 13 and Hartley guinea pigs are highly susceptible, Strain 2 and Magnum animals were found to be relatively resistent (Stone et al. 1969; Madrid et al. 1981b). In addition, in outbred animal strains like Hartley guinea pigs the incidence of chronic EAE and the clinical course of the disease is variable when the animals are obtained from different breeders. The main clinical data from our experiments with Strain 13 and Hartley guinea pigs from different sources are summarized in Table 1.

Table 1. Chronic relapsing EAE in different strains of guinea pigs

	Strain 13	Hartley New Springville	FIV
Number of animals	119	57	55
Acute EAE incidence	83 %	81 %	96 %
Acute EAE mortality	13 %	49 %	33 %
Chronic EAE incidence	81 %	43 %	62 %
Relapses incidence	79 %	32 %	43 %
Mean relapse	40 days	35 days	23 days
interval	(30–90)	(8–65)	(7–90)

All animals were sensitized with 50 mg Hartley guinea pig spinal cord tissue and 2 mg myobacterium in the adjuvant; inoculation site: dorsum of the hind legs

114

Following sensitization according to the method described by Wisniewski and Keith (1977), Strain 13 animals have a low mortality rate during the acute stage of the disease and a large proportion of the animals develop a chronic disease course with several relapses and remissions. Eighty-three percent of the animals suffer from acute EAE (10–20 dps), which is followed by a remission with complete clinical recovery in the majority of the animals. The first relapse of the disease is generally noted between the 40th and 100th day after sensitization and is then followed by further exacerbations and remissions of the disease. Active demyelinating disease has been noted in Strain 13 animals up to 15 months after sensitization; relapses which occur after 1 year, however, are relatively mild and short lasting.

In Hartley guinea pigs the disease course is more variable than in Strain 13 animals. In general Hartley guinea pigs are affected more severely during the acute disease episode, which results in a high mortality during this stage of the disease. Also during the early chronic disease stage (40–100 dps) Hartley guinea pigs suffer from more severe disease than Strain 13 animals. This results in a relatively high mortality also during this stage of the disease, in the presence of high grade of neurological deficit in the surviving animals and in very large demyelinated lesions in the central nervous system. On the other hand, the overall disease duration in Hartley guinea pigs is shorter than in Strain 13 animals; the last active relapses of the disease were noted between 6–9 months after sensitization.

As Hartley guinea pigs are not an inbred strain of animals, pronounced variation in the disease course may be noted when animals are obtained from different breeders. This can be seen in Table 1 in a comparison between Hartley guinea pigs obtained from New Springville Laboratoy Animals (NY) and from the Forschungsinstitut für Versuchstierzucht (Himberg, Austria). Differences concern mainly the incidence of chronic EAE and the incidence of relapses. Furthermore, the interval between individual relapses in Hartley guinea pigs obtained from FIV – frequently not more than 10–20 days – is in general shorter than that in animals obtained from New Springville Lab. Animals and Strain 13 guinea pigs. This, however, results in a less clear-cut clinicopathological correlation of exacerbations and remissions than in animals with long intervals between individual relapses.

Another difference between different strains of guinea pigs is related to lesional topography. Whereas in Strain 13 and Hartley guinea pigs from New Springville Lab. Animals the majority of large demyelinated plaques is located in the spinal cord, nearly all Hartley guinea pigs from FIV have extensive lesions in the centrum semiovale. In this strain of animals lesions may even be entirely localized in the brain hemispheres with only a few inflammatory cuffs in the spinal cord and brain stem. In such a strain of animals, studies dealing with the pathogenesis of relapses must be controlled in detail by pathohistology, since the majority of lesions in the centrum semiovale are clinically silent.

To summarize, Strain 13 animals are most suitable for the study of mechanisms leading to relapses of the disease. On the other hand, Hartley guinea pigs are superior for the study of the pathogenesis of demyelination since myelin destruction in chronic EAE is much more extensive in this animal strain than in Strain 13 animals.

6.2.2 Antigen Dose

As has already been noted by others, the dose of the antigen used for sensitization influences the expression of chronic relapsing EAE (Keith and McDermott 1980). In Hartley guinea pigs a dose of 50–75 mg spinal cord tissue and 2–3 mg mycobacterium in the adjuvant is most effective in the induction of chronic relapsing EAE (Fig. 34, Table 2). A lower dose results in a high mortality in the acute stage of the disease (10–20 dps). Although the acute mortality was low after sensitization with 100 mg of spinal cord tissue, all animals died early in the subacute stage of the disease (20–40 dps). A similar high mortality in the subacute stage of the disease was noted by Keith and McDermott (1980), when Hartley guinea pigs were sensitized with 100 mg spinal cord tissue in the dorsum of front and hind legs.

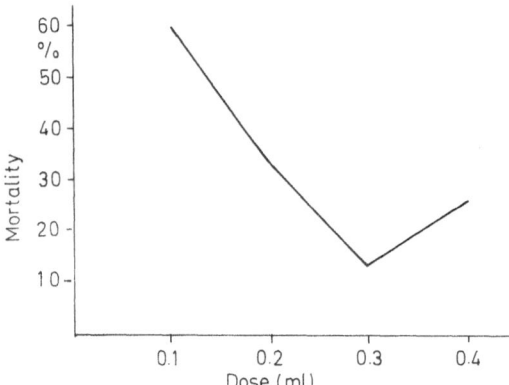

Fig. 34. Effect of antigen dose on acute mortality in chronic relapsing EAE. Hartley guinea pigs (FIV, Himberg, Austria) were sensitized 14–21 days after birth into the dorsum of the hind legs (0.1–0.2 ml emulsion) or the dorsum of the hind legs and the nuchal area (0.3–0.4 ml emulsion). 0.1 ml of the emulsion contained 25 mg Hartley guinea pig spinal cord tissue, 0.025 ml saline, 0.05 ml CFA, and 1 mg heat-inactivated myobacterium

Table 2. Effect of antigen dose on the clinical course of chronic EAE (Hartley GP; FIV, Himberg, Austria)

Antigen dose	Number of animals	Acute EAE		Chronic disease severity		
		Incidence	Severity	Subacute	Early chronic	Late chronic
0.2	55	96 %	3.22	2.65	2.8	2.75
0.3	27	85 %	2.48	2.5	2.6	2.8

0.1 ml antigen contained 25 mg Hartley guinea pig spinal cord tissue, 0.025 ml saline, 0.05 ml CFA, and 1 mg heat-inactivated mycobacterium

116

Within the range of 25–75 mg spinal cord tissue in the sensitization medium, the severity and mortality during the acute disease episode is mainly affected (Fig. 34, Table 2). With increasing antigen dose the disease becomes less severe during the acute stage and a higher proportion of animals develop chronic progressive or chronic relapsing EAE. Although a comparison between different animal strains is difficult, the high dose of antigen used for sensitization by Stone and Lerner (1965) may be responsible for the low incidence of an acute disease episode in this model.

6.2.3 Age of the Animals at the Time of Sensitization

As has already been shown, the age of the animals at the time of sensitization is of critical importance for the induction of chronic relapsing EAE (Stone and Lerner 1965; Lassmann and Wisniewski 1979b). In Hartley guinea pigs the mortality during the acute stage of the disease rises sharply, when animals are sensitized later than 28 days after birth (Fig. 35). Whereas animals sensitized between 14 and 21 days after birth showed the highest incidence of chronic relapsing EAE, animals challenged earlier during life more frequently developed a chronic progressive disease course (Lassmann and Wisniewski 1979b).

It must be stressed however, that the young age of animals is not necessarily required for the induction of chronic EAE. As will be discussed in detail below, chronic EAE in less susceptible animals like Sprague Dawley rats is mainly found when young adults are challenged with CNS tissue.

6.2.4 Inoculation Site

In the present experiments all animals were sensitized by the injection of the antigen into the dorsum of the hind legs. When higher antigen doses than 50 mg spinal cord tissue were used, additional inoculum was injected into the nuchal area.

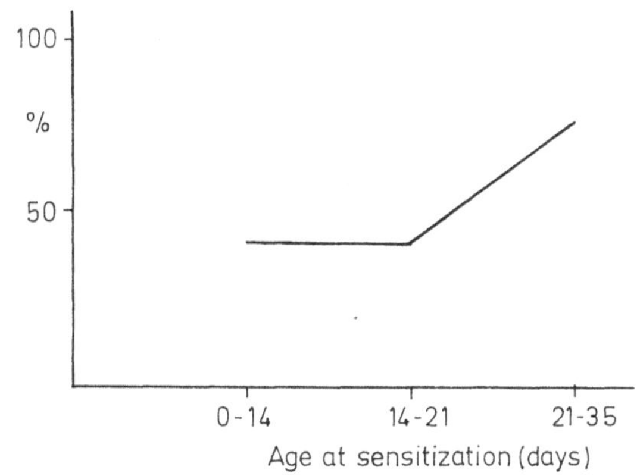

Fig. 35. Acute mortality of Hartley guinea pigs sensitized at different ages. Hartley guinea pigs (New Springville Lab. Animals) sensitized with 50 mg Hartley guinea pig spinal cord in CFA with additional 2 mg heat-inactivated mycobacterium into the dorsum of both hind legs

Comparing the present results with those published earlier by others (Stone and Lerner 1965; Keith and McDermott 1980), it can be extrapolated that challenge into the hind legs augments mainly the expression of the disease during the acute stage (10–20 dps). Inoculation into the nuchal area in the same animal strain and with the same antigen dose results in a more protracted disease course with only low disease incidence during the acute stage of the disease (Keith and McDermott 1980).

6.2.5 Amount of Mycobacterium in the Adjuvant

Chronic EAE with extensive demyelination is induced in small rodents only when a high amount of mycobacterium is added to the inoculum (Stone and Lerner 1965; Wisniewski and Keith 1977; Keith and McDermott 1980). When the amount of mycobacterium is reduced in the sensitization medium, juvenile guinea pigs challenged with a high dose of CNS antigen develop a lower incidence of acute as well as chronic disease, and in general the size of the lesions is smaller. It is at present not known why such a high dose of mycobacterium is needed for the induction of chronic demyelinating EAE. However, induction of an immune response against lipid hapten of myelin, which may be involved in the pathogenesis of demyelination, also requires the presence of high amounts of mycobacterium in the adjuvant (Niedieck 1975; Niedieck and Lohmann 1981).

6.2.6 Spinal Cord Subfractions

A high incidence of chronic demyelinating EAE has so far only been induced when native guinea pig spinal cord was used as antigen for sensitization (Wisniewski et al. 1980a; Wisniewski et al. 1982). Sensitization with a comparable dose of purified myelin increases the mortality during the acute stage of EAE and decreases the incidence of chronic demylinating EAE (Madrid et al. 1981a). Pretreatment of spinal cord tissue with lipid solvents prior to sensitization further decreases the incidence of EAE and demyelination (Schwerer et al. 1981a; Madrid et al. 1981a). Sensitization of juvenile guinea pigs with myelin basic protein (250 μg and 2 mg mycobacterium in the adjuvant) induced acute EAE with high mortality (Wisniewski et al. 1980). Some of the remaining animals developed a mild chronic leukoencephalitis, which was clinically silent in the majority of the animals. Plaque-like demyelination was not noted after MBP sensitization. Panitch and Ciccone (1981) described a chronic relapsing form of EAE following sensitization with MBP; pathohistologically a chronic leukoencephalomyelitis with little demyelination was found. Sensitization of guinea pigs with MBP together with myelin lipids resulted in a low incidence of chronic demyelinating EAE (Madrid et al. 1981).

6.2.7 Chronic EAE in Sprague Dawley Rats

For induction of chronic EAE in Sprague Dawley rats young adult animals (200–250 g body wt.) were sensitized with 50 mg guinea pig spinal cord in adjuvant with an increased amount of mycobacterium, a mixture identical to that used for induction of chronic relapsing EAE in guinea pigs. The inoculum was injected into the dorsum of the hind legs.

Clinically the majority of the animals (57%) developed a chronic relapsing disease course with an acute disease episode (10–25 dps) followed by recovery and a further exacerbation of the disease between the 40th and 100th day after sensitization (Fig. 36); the other animals either showed a progressive disease course (10%) or suffered only from a single acute or chronic disease episode.

The age of the animals at the time of sensitization clinically affected mainly the disease severity during the acute stage of the disease (Fig. 37); with increasing age of the animals at the time of sensitization the acute disease became more severe and lasted longer.

Pathohistologically a complex pattern of alterations in the CNS and PNS was noted. The acute episode was characterized by exclusive disease of the central nervous system. The cerebellar white matter was regularly affected followed by the order of incidence by the spinal cord and the centrum semiovale. CNS disease started with perivenous inflammation. The extent of demyelination increased with time after sensitization, reaching its maximum with large confluent plaques 30–40 dps. During the following weeks the extent of active demyelination in the CNS lesions decreased and remyelination of the plaques occurred.

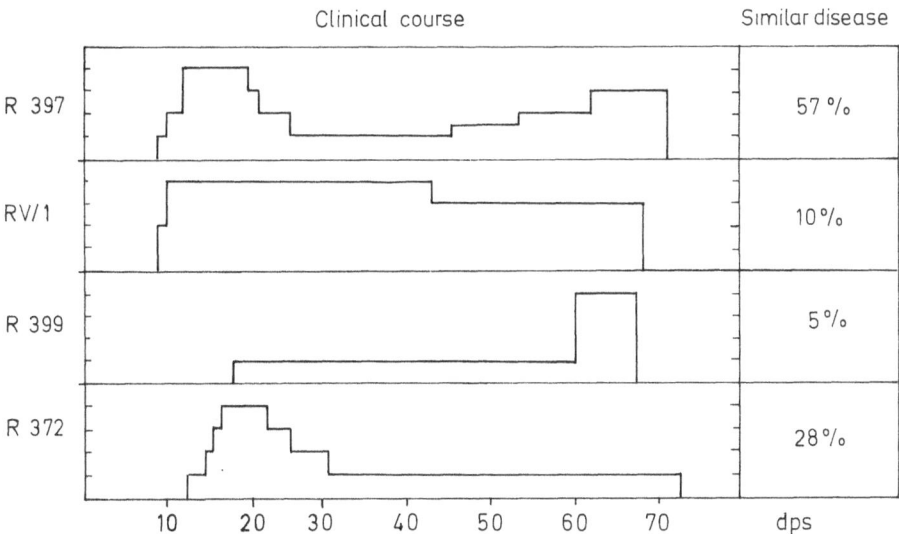

Fig. 36. Chronic EAE in Sprague Dawley rats. Each clinical course was obtained from a single animal. On the *right* the incidence (%) of animals with similar clinical disease is given. Twenty-one young adult animals (200–300 g) were sensitized with 50 mg Hartley guinea pig spinal cord tissue as described in the text

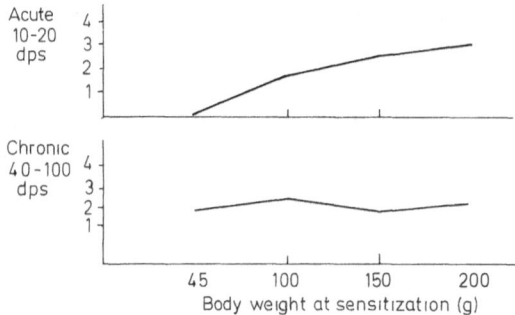

Acute
10-20
dps

Chronic
40-100
dps

Body weight at sensitization (g)

Fig. 37. Chronic EAE in Sprague Dawley rats. Mean disease severity in animals sensitized at various times after birth. The clinical severity represents the average maximal clinical scores reached by the animals either during the acute (10–20 dps) or the chronic stage (40–100 dps) of the disease. The age of the animals at the time of sensitization is indicated by the body weight of the animals

The second clinical episode of the disease (40–100 dps) was due mainly to lesions restricted to the peripheral nervous system. Lesions in the PNS were either predominantly inflammatory (Fig. 28a,b) or accompanied by extensive demyelination (Fig. 28c,d). PNS disease in the chronic stage was similar regardless of the age of the animals at the time of sensitization. CNS involvement, however, was absent, when newborn animals (45 g body wt.) were sensitized. With increasing age at the time of sensitization, CNS lesions became more frequent and extensive.

6.2.8 Conclusions

The induction of chronic demyelinating EAE is difficult, and many different factors seem to play a role in the expression of chronic CNS and PNS disease.

Two aspects in the sensitization procedure are common for all the above-mentioned models of chronic EAE. They are the high dose of antigen and the high dose of mycobacterium in the adjuvant. One possible explanation for these requirements may be that overloading of the immune response with antigens may induce some kind of tolerance responsible for suppression of acute EAE.

The juvenile age of the animals at the time of sensitization does not seem to be an absolute requirement for induction of chronic EAE. It is necessary in highly susceptible animal strains like guinea pigs. However, in more EAE-resistant animals like Sprague Dawley rats the highest incidence of chronic CNS disease was noted when young adult animals were sensitized. Thus the induction of chronic EAE seems to be dependent upon several variables, including the maturity of the immune system, the susceptibility of animal strains for EAE, and the relative dose of antigen and adjuvant per unit body weight.

Only minor variations in the preparation and the dose of the antigen and adjuvant and in the selection of the sensitization site may change the clinical course and pathohistological expression of chronic EAE dramatically. It thus seems to be necessary that the model of chronic EAE used in the experiments must be standar-

120

dized clinically and pathohistologically before starting immunological and neuro-chemical studies.

Acknowledgments

We are greatly indebted to Prof. F. Seitelberger and Prof. Dr. H.M. Wisniewski for helpful discussion. We would also like to thank Mrs. M. Leiszer, Ms. A. Cervenka, and Ms. U. Juszczak for skillful technical assistance and photographic work, and Ms. F. Friedrich for her patience and excellent secretarial assistence.

The study was funded in part by the Fonds zur Förderung der wissenschaftlichen Forschung, Austria, Project S-25/07.

7 References

Abramsky O (1979) Immunological studies of isolated oligodendrocytes in relation to multiple sclerosis. In: Rose FC (ed) Clinical Neuroimmunology. Blackwell, Oxford, pp 344–353

Ackermann HP, Ulrich J, Heitz PV (1981) Experimental allergic encephalomyelitis: exsudate and cellular infiltrates in the spinal cord of Lewis rats. Acta Neuropathol 54:149–152

Adams CWM (1975) The onset and progression of the lesion in multiple sclerosis. J Neurol Sci 25:165–182

Adams CWM (1977) Pathology of multiple sclerosis: progression of the lesion. Br Med Bull 33:15–20

Adams RD, Kubik CS (1952) The morbid anatomy of the demyelating diseases. Am J Med 12:510–546

Adams RD, Cammermeyer J, Denny-Brown D (1948) Acute necrotising haemorrhagic encephalopathy. J Neuropathol Exp Neurol 8:1–29

Agrawal HC, Hartman BK, Shearer WT, Kalmback S, Margolis FG (1977) Purification and immunohistochemical localization of rat brain proteolipid protein. J Neurochem 28:495–508

Aita JF, Bennet DR, Anderson RE, Ziter F (1978) Cranial CT appearance of acute multiple sclerosis. Neurology 28:251-255

Allen IV, Mc Keown SR (1979), A histological, histochemical and biochemical study of the macroscopically normal white matter in multiple sclerosis. J Neurol Sci 41:81-91

Allen IV, Glover G, McKeown SR, McCormick D (1979), The cellular origin of lysosomal enzymes in the plaque in multiple sclerosis. II. A histochemical study with combined demonstration of myelin and acid phosphatase. Neuropathol Appl Neurobiol 5:197–210

Allen IV, Glover G, Anderson R (1981), Abnormalities in the macroscopically normal white matter in cases of mild or spinal multiple sclerosis (MS). Acta Neuropathol [Suppl] VII:176–178

Alvord EC (1970) Acute disseminated encephalomyelitis and "allergic" neuroencephalopathies. In: Vinken PI, Bruyn GW (eds) Handbook of clinical neurology, vol. 9. Elsevier, New York, pp 500–571

Alvord EC Jr (1980) Chronic relapsing experimental allergic encephalomyelitis induced in monkeys with myelin basic protein. J Neuropathol Exp Neurol 39:338

Alvord EC Jr, Shaw CM, Hruby S, Kies M.W. (1979) Has myelin basic protein received a fair trial in the treatment of multiple sclerosis. Ann Neurol 6:461–468

Andrews JM (1972), The ultrastructural neuropathology of multiple sclerosis. In: Wolfgram F, Ellison GW, Stevens JG (eds) Multiple sclerosis. Immunology, virology and ultrastructure. Academic, New York, pp 23–52

Anton G, Wohlwill Fr (1912) Multiple nicht eitrige Enzephalomyelitis und multiple Sklerose. Z gesamt Neurol Psychiatr 12:31–98

Appel SH, Bornstein MB (1964) The application of tissue culture to the study of experimental allergic encephalomyelitis. II. Serum factors, responsible for demyelination. J exp Med 119:303–312

Arnason BGW, Winkler GF, Hadler NM (1969) Cell mediated demyelination of peripheral nerve in culture. Lab Invest 21:1–10

Arnon R, Crisp E, Kelley R, Ellison GW, Myers LM, Tourtelotte WW (1980) Antiganglioside antibodies in multiple sclerosis. J Neurol Sci 46:179–186

Aström KE, Waksman BH (1962) The passive transfer of experimental allergic encephalomyelitis and neuritis with living lymph node cells. J Pathol Bacteriol 83:89–106

Auff E, Budka H (1980) Immunohistologische Methoden in der Neuropathologie. In: Jellinger K, Gross H (eds) Current topics in neuropathology, vol 6. Facultas, Wien, pp 21–30

Baker AB (1943) Guillain-Barré's disease (encephalo-myelo-radiculitis). A review of 33 cases. Lancet 63:384-398

Baló J (1928) Encephalitis periaxialis concentrica. Arch Neurol 19:242-264

Becker NH, Hirano A Zimmermann HM (1968) Observations of the distribution of exogenous peroxidase in the rat cerebrum. J Neuropathol Exp Neurol 27:439–452

122

Bernard CCA (1976) Experimental autoimmune encephalomyelitis in mice: genetic control of susceptibility. J Immunogenet 3:263–274

Bernard CCA, Carnegie PR (1975) Experimental autoimmune encephalomyelitis in mice: immunologic response to mouse spinal cord and myelin basic proteins. J Immunol 114:1537–1540

Blakemore WF (1973) Remyelination in the superior cerebellar peduncle in the mouse following demyelination induced by feeding cuprizone. J Neurol Sci 20:73-85

Blakemore WF (1975) Remyelination by Schwann cells of axons demyelinated by intraspinal injection of 6-aminonicotinamide in the rat. J Neurocytol 4:745–757

Blakemore WF (1976) Invasion of Schwann cells into the spinal cord following local injection of lysolecithin. Neuropathol appl Neurobiol 2:21–39

Blakemore WF, Paterson RC (1975) Observations on the interactions of Schwann cells and astrocytes following X-irradiation of neonatal rat spinal cord. J Neurocytol 4:573-585

Bornstein MB, Appel SH (1961) The application of tissue culture to the study of experimental "allergic" encephalomyelitis. I. Patterns of demyelination. J Neuropathol Exp Neurol 20:141–147

Bornstein MB, Appel SH (1965) Tissue culture studies of demyelination. Ann NY Acad Sci 122:280–286

Bornstein MB, Raine CS (1970) Experimental allergic encephalomyelitis: antiserum inhibition of myelination in vitro. Lab Invest 23:536-542

Bornstein MB, Iwanami H (1971) Experimental allergic encephalomyelitis: demyelinating activity of serum and sensitised lymphe node cells on cultured nerve tissue. J Neuropathol Exp Neurol 30:240–248

Brett M, Weller RO (1978) Intracellular serum proteins in cerebral gliomas and metastatic tumors: an immunoperoxidase study. Neuropathol Appl Neurobiol 4:263–272

Brightman MW (1965) The distribution within the brain of ferritin injected into the cerebrospinal fluid compartments. Part 2 (Parenchymal distribution). Am J Anat 117:193–220

Brightman MW (1977) The morphology of blood brain interfaces. Exp Eye Res [Suppl] 1–25

Brightman MW, Klatzo I, Olsson Y, Reese TS (1970) The blood brain barrier to proteins under normal and pathological conditions. J Neurol Sci 10:215–239

Broman T (1964) Blood brain barrier damage in multiple sclerosis. Supra-vital test observations. Acta Neurol Scand [Suppl] 10:21-24

Brosnan CF, Stoner GL, Bloom BR, Wisniewski HM (1977) Studies on demylination by activated lymphocytes in the rabbit eye. II. Antibody dependent cell mediated demyelination. J Immunol 118:2103–2110

Brostoff SW, Powers JM (1975) Allergic encephalomyelitis: modification of the response by synthetic membrane structures containing bovine myeline basic protein and cerebroside. Brain Res 93:175–181

Brown AM, McFarlin DE, Raine CS (1981) Chronic relapsing EAE in the mouse. J Neuropathol Exp Neurol 40:320

Bubis JJ, Luse SA (1964) An electron microscopic study of experimental allergic encephalomyelitis in the rat. Am J Pathol 44:299–317

Bunge MB, Bunge RP, Ris H (1961) Ultrastructural study of remyelination in an experimental lesion in adult cat spinal cord. J Biophys Biochem Cytol 10:67–74

Burks JS, Devald-MacMillan B, Jankovsky L, Gerdes J (1979) Characterization of coronarviruses isolated using multiple sclerosis autopsy brain material. Neurology 29:547

Cammer W, Bloom BR, Norton WT, Gordon S (1978) Degradation of basic protein in myelin by neutral proteases secreted by stimulated macrophages: a possible mechanism of inflammatory demyelination. Proc Natl Acad Sci USA 75:1554–1558

Carp R, Licursi PC, Merz PA, Merz GS (1972) Decreased percentage of polymorphonuclear neutrophils in mouse peripheral blood after inoculation of material from multiple sclerosis patients. J Exp Med 136:618–629

Caspary EA (1977) Humoral factors involved in immune processes in multiple sclerosis and allergic encephalomyelitis. Br Med Bull 33:50–53

Charcot JM (1868) Histologie de la sclerose en plaque. Gaz Hôpital (Paris) 41:554-566

Colover J (1980) A new pattern of spinal-cord demyelination in guinea pigs with acute experimental allergic encephalomyelitis mimicking multiple sclerosis. Br J Exp Pathol 61:390-400

Cook RD, Wisniewski HM (1973) The role of oligodendroglia and astroglia in Wallerian degeneration of the optic nerve. Brain Res 61:191–206

Cook SD, Dowling PC (1981) The role of autoantibodies and immune complexes in the pathogenesis of Guillain-Barré syndrome. Ann Neurol [Suppl] 9:70–79

Courville CB (1970) Concentric sclerosis. In: Vinken PJ, Bruyn GW (eds) Handbook of clinical neurology, vol 9. Elsevier, New York, pp 437–451

Cutler RWP, Devel RK, Barlow CF (1967) Albumin exchange between plasma and cerebrospinal fluid. Arch Neurol 17:261–270

Cuzner ML, Davison AN (1979) The scientific basis of multiple sclerosis. In: Baum H, Gergely J (eds) Molecular aspects of medicine, vol 2. Pergamon, New York, p 147

Dal Canto MC, Rabinowitz SG (1982) Experimental models of virus-induced demyelination in the central nervous system. Ann Neurol 11:109–127

Dal Canto MC, Wisniewski HM, Johnson AB, Brostoff SW, Raine CS (1975) Vesicular disruption of myelin in autoimmune demyelination. J Neurol Sci 24:313–319

Dal Canto MC, Rabinowitz SG, Johnson AB (1979) Virus induced demyelination. Production by viral temperature-sensitive mutant. J. Neurol. Sci 42:155–168

Daniel PM, Lam DKC, Pratt OE (1981) Changes in the effectiveness of the blood brain and blood spinal cord barriers in experimental allergic encephalomyelitis. Possible relevance to multiple sclerosis. J Neurol Sci 52:211–219

Dawson JW (1916) The histology of disseminated sclerosis. Trans R Soc 50:517–740

De Preux J, Mair WGP (1974) Ultrastructure of optic nerve in Schilder's disease, Devic's disease and disseminated sclerosis. Acta Neuropathol 30:225–242

Dévic C (1894) Myélite subaigue compliquée de névrite optique. Bull Med 8:1033

Dinkler (1904) Zur Kasuistik der multiplen Herdsklerose des Gehirns und Rückenmarks. Dtsch Z Nervenheilk 26:233–247

Dowling PC, Kim SU, Murray MR, Cook SD (1968) Serum 19 S and 7 S demyelinating antibodies in multiple sclerosis. J Immunol 101:1101–1104

Dubois-Dalq M, Niedieck B, Buyse M (1970) Action of anticerebroside sera on myelinated nervous tissue cultures. Pathologica 5:331–347

Dubois-Dalq M Schumacher G, Worthington EK (1975), Immunoperoxidase studies on multiple sclerosis brain. Neurology 25:496

Edvinson L, McKenzie ET (1977) Amine mechanisms in the cerebral circulation. Pharmacol Rev 28:275–348

Ehrlich P (1885) Das Sauerstoff-Bedürfnis des Organismus. Eine farbenanalytische Studie. Hirschwald, Berlin

Eickhoff K, Wikström J, Poser S, Bauer H (1977) Protein profile of cerebrospinal fluid in multiple sclerosis with special reference to the function of the blood brain barrier. J Neurol 214:207–215

Esiri MM (1977) Immunoglobulin containing cells in multiple sclerosis plaques. Lancet 2:478–480

Feasby TE, Hahn AF, Gilbert JJ (1980) Passive transfer of demyelinating activity in Guillain-Barré polyneuropathy. Neurology 30:363

Feigin I, Popoff N (1966) Regeneration of myelin in multiple sclerosis. Neurology 16: 364–372

Felgenhauer K (1974) Protein size and cerebrospinal fluid composition. Klin Wochenschr 52:1158–1164

Ferraro A, Cazzullo CL (1948) Chronic experimental allergic encephalomyelitis in monkeys. J Neuropathol Exp Neurol 7:235–260

Field EJ (1967) The significance of astroglial hypertrophy in scrapie, Kuru, multiple sclerosis and old age, together with a note on the possible nature of the scrapie agent. Dtsch Z Nervenklinik 192:265–274

Field EJ (1979) Multiple sclerosis: recent advances in aethiopathogenesis. In: Smith WT, Cavanagh JB (eds) Recent advances in neuropathology I. Churchill, Livingstone, London, pp 277–298

Field EJ, Raine CS (1964) Examination of multiple sclerosis biopsy specimens, 3rd European regional conference on electron microscopy. Czechoslovak Academy of Sciences, Prague, p 289

Field EJ, Raine CS (1969) Experimental allergic encephalomyelitis: an electron microscopic study. Am J Path 49:537–553

Field EJ, Miller H, Russel DS (1962) Observations on glial inclusion bodies in a case of acute disseminated sclerosis. J Clin Pathol 15:278–284

Field EJ, Cowshall S, Narang HK, Bell TM (1972) Viruses in multiple sclerosis. Lancet II:280–281

Finkelnburg (1901), Über Myeloencephalitis disseminata und Sclerosis multiplex acuta mit anatomischem Befund. Dtsch Z Nervenheilk 20:408–425

Fog T (1950) Topographic distribution of plaques in the spinal cord in multiple sclerosis Arch Neurol 63:382–414

Fontana A, Grieder A, Arrenbrecht St, Grob P (1980a) In vitro stimulation of glia cells by a lymphocyte produced factor. J Neurol Sci 46:55–62

Fontana A, Grieder A, Jost R, Balsiger S, Grob PJ (1980b) Glia stimulating factor: Further analysis of secretion mechanisms. Allergol Immunopathol 8:454

124

Fraenkel M, Jakob A (1913) Zur Pathologie der multiplen Sklerose mit besonderer Berücksichtigung der akuten Formen Z. Neurol. 14:565–603

Freund J, Lipton MM, Morrison LR (1950) Demyelination in the guinea pig in chronic allergic encephalomyelitis. Produced by injecting guinea pig brain in oil emulsion containing a variant of mycobacterium butyricum. Arch Pathol 50:108–121

Frick E (1969) Zur Pathogenese entzündlicher Nervenkrankheiten: Über die Bedeutung immunokompetenter Zellen. Fortschr Med 87:1191–1194

Frick E (1979) Immunologie des Demyelinisierungsprozesses. In: Schmidt RM (ed) Multiple Sklerose, Epidemiologie, Immunologie, Ultrastruktur. VEB Fischer, Jena, pp 167–259

Frick E, Scheid-Seydel L (1958) Untersuchungen mit J^{131}-markiertem Albumin über Austauschvorgänge zwischen Plasma und Liquor cerebrospinalis. Klin Wochenschr 36:66–69

Friede RL (1961) Enzyme histochemical studies in multiple sclerosis. Arch Neurol 5:103–113

Friedemann U, Elkeles A (1934) The blood brain barrier in infectious diseases: its permeability to toxins in relation to their electrical charges. Lancet 226:719–724

Ghatak NR, Hirano A, Doron Y, Zimmmerman HH (1973) Remyelination in multiple sclerosis with peripheral type myelin. Arch Neurol 29:262–267

Gledhill RF, McDonald WI (1977) Morphological characteristics of central demyelination and remyelination; a single fiber study. Ann Neurol 1:552–560

Gledhill RF, Harrison BM, McDonald WI (1973) Demyelination and remyelination after acute spinal cord compression. Exp Neurol 38:472–487

Goldmann EE (1913) Vitalfärbung am Zentralnervensystem. Beitrag zur Physiopathologie des Plexus chorioideus und der Hirnhäute. In: Abhandlungen der Königlichen Preußischen Akademie der Wissenschaften. Physikalisch-mathematische Klasse, vol 1. Berlin, pp 1–60

Gonatas NK (1970) Ultrastructural observations in a case of multiple sclerosis. J. Neuropathol Exp Neurol 19:149

Gonsette R, André-Balisaux G (1965) La permeabilité de vaisseaux cérébraux. Partie 4 (Etude des lésions de la barriére hémato-encéphalique dans la sclérose en plaques). Acta Neurol Psychiat Belg 65:19–34

Greenfield S, Brostoff S, Eylar EH, Morell P (1973) Protein comparison of myelin of the peripheral nervous system. J Neurochem 20:1207–1216

Gross PM, Teasdale GM, Angerson WJ, Harper AM, (1981) H^2-receptors mediate increases of permeability of the blood-brain barrier during arterial histamine infusion. Brain Res 210: 396–400

Grundke-Iqbal I, Bornstein MB (1980) Multiple sclerosis: serum gamma globulin and demyelination in culture. Neurology 30:749–754

Grundke-Iqbal I, Lassmann H, Wisniewski HM (1980) Chronic relapsing experimental allergic encephalomyelitis. Immunohistochemical studies. Arch Neurol 37:651–656

Grundke-Iqbal I, Raine CS, Johnson AB, Brosnan CF, Bornstein MB (1981) Experimental allergic encephalomyelitis. Characterisation of serum factors causing demyelination and swelling of myelin. J Neurol Sci 50:63–79

Gudnadóttir M, Helgadóttir H, Bjarnason O, Jónsdóttir K (1964) Virus isolated from the brain of a patient with multiple sclerosis. Exp Neurol 9:85–95

Guseo A, Jellinger K (1975) The signilficance of perivascular infiltrations in multiple sclerosis. Neurol 211:51–60

Gyldensted C (1976) Computer tomography of the cerebrum in multiple sclerosis. Neuroradiology 12:33–42

Hallervorden J (1940) Die zentralen Entmarkungserkrankungen. Dtsch Z Nervenheilk 150:201–239

Hallpike JF, Adams CWM (1969) Proteolysis and myelin breakdown; a review of recent histochemical and biochemical studies. Histochem J 1:559–578

Hallpike JF, Adams CWM, Bayliss OB (1970) Histochemistry of myelin. Proteolysis of normal myelin and release of lipid by extracts of degenerating nerve. Histochem J 2:315–321

Hashim GA, Wood DA, Moscarello MA (1980) Myelin lipophilin-induced experimental allergic encephalomyelitis in guinea pigs. Progress in clinical and biological research. Neurochem Clin Neurol 39:21–39

Hasson J, Terry RD, Zimmerman HM (1958) Peripheral neuropathy in multiple sclerosis. Neurology 8:503–510

Hauw JJ, Escourolle R (1977) Filaments and multilammellated cytoplasmic inclusions in progressive multifocal leukoencephalopathy. Acta Neuropathol 37:263–265

Haymaker W, Kernohan JW (1949) The Laundry-Guillain-Barré syndrome, a clinico-pathological report of fifty fatal cases and a critique of the literature . Medicine 28:59–141

Henschen SE (1896) Akute disseminierte Rückenmarkssklerose mit Neuritis nach Diphtherie bei einem Kinde. Fortschr Med 14:529–550

Herndon RM, Griffin DE, McCormick U, Weiner LP (1975) Mouse hepatitis virus induced recurrent demyelination: a preliminary report. Arch Neurol 32:32–35

Hirano A, Levine S, Zimmerman HM (1968) Remyelination in the central nervous system after cyanide intoxication. J Neuropathol Exp Neurol 27:234–245

Hirano A, Dembitzer HM, Becker NH, Levine S, Zimmerman HM (1970) Fine structural alterations of the blood brain barrier in experimental allergic encephalomyelitis. J Neuropathol Exp Neurol 29:432–440

Hochwald GM (1970) Influx of serum proteins and their concentration in the spinal fluid along the neuraxis. J Neurol Sci 10:269–278

Hughes D, Field EJ (1967) Myelinotoxicity of serum and spinal fluid in multiple sclerosis: a critical assessment. Clin Exp Immunol 2:295–309

Hurst EW (1941) Acute haemorrhagic leucoencephalitis. A previously undefined entity. Med J Aust 2:1–6

Ibrahim MZM, Adams CWM (1963) The relationship between enzyme activity and neuroglia in plaques of multiple sclerosis. J Neurol Neurosurg Psychiatry 26:101–110

Ibrahim MZM, Adams CWM (1965) The relations between enzyme activity and neuroglia in early plaques of multiple sclerosis. J Pathol Bacteriol 90:239–243

Itoyama Y, Sternberger NH, Webster H de F, Quarles RH, Cohen SR, Richardson EP (1980) Immunocytochemical observations on the distribution of myelin-associated glycoprotein and myelin basic protein in multiple sclerosis lesions. Ann Neurol 7:167–177

Jacob H (1948) Zur hirnpathologischen Diagnose des akuten und chronisch rezidivierenden Hirnödems. Arch Psychiatr Nervenkr 179:158–163

Jankovic B, Draskoci M, Janjic M (1965) Passive transfer of "allergic" encephalomyelitis with anti brain serum, injected into the lateral ventricle of the brain. Nature 207: 428–429

Jellinger K (1969) Einige morphologische Aspekte der Multiplen Sklerose. Wien Z Nervenheilk [Suppl] II:12–37

Jellinger K, Seitelberger F (1958) Akute tödliche Entmarkungsenzephalitis nach wiederholten Hirntrockenzellinjektionen. Klin Wochenschr 36:437–441

Jervis GA, Koprowski H (1948) Experimental allergic encephalomyelitis. J Neuropathol Exp Neurol 7:309–320

Jochwed B (1925) Ein Fall einer Erkrankung des Nervensystems im Verlaufe der Schutzimpfungen gegen Wut. Z Gesamt Neurol Psychiatr 41:583

Karcher D, Lassmann H, Lowenthal A, Kitz K, Wisniewski HM (1982) Antibodies-restricted heterogeneity in serum and cerebrospinal fluid of chronic relapsing experimental allergic encephalomyelitis. J Neuroimmunol 2:93–106

Karpiak SE, Graf L, Rapport MM (1976) Antiserum to brain gangliosides produces recurrent epileptiform activity. Science 194: 735–737

Keith AB, McDermott JR (1980) Optimum conditions for inducing chronic relapsing experimental allergic encephalomyelitis in guinea pigs. J Neurol Sci 46:353–364

Ketelaer CJ, Lervitte A, Perier O (1966) Histopathologie de la moette lumbo-sacrée et de la queue de cheval dans une série de cas vérifiés de sclerose. Acta Neurol Scand 42:33–51

Kies MW, Murphy JB, Alvord EC (1960) Fractionation of guinea pig brain proteins with encephalitogenic activity. Fed Proc 19:207

Kim SU, Murray MR, Tourtellotte WW (1970) Demonstration in tissue culture of myelino-toxicity in cerebrospinal fluid and brain extracts from multiple sclerosis patients. J Neuropathol Exp Neurol 29:420–431

Kirk J (1979) The fine structure of the CNS in multiple sclerosis. II. Vesicular demyelination in an acute case. Neuropathol Appl Neurobiol 5:289–294

Kitz K, Lassmann H, Wisniewski HM (1981) Isolated leptomeninges of the spinal cord: an ideal tool to study inflammatory reaction in EAE. Acta Neuropathol [Suppl] 7:179–181

Klatzo I, Miquel J, Ferris PJ, Prokop JD, Smith DE (1964) Observations on the passage of fluorescein labelled serum proteins (FLSP) from the cerebrospinal fluid. J Neuropathol Exp Neurol 23:18–35

Koestner A, McCullough B, Krakowka GS, Long JF, Olsen RG (1974) Canine distemper, a virus induced demyelinating encephalitis. In: Zeman W, Lenette EH (eds) Slow virus diseases. Williams and Wilkins, Baltimore, pp 86–101

Kosunen TU, Waksman BH, Samuelsson K (1963) Radioautographic study of cellular mechanisms in delayed hypersensitivity. II. Experimental allergic encephalomyelitis in the rat. J Neuropathol Exp Neurol 22:367–380

126

Krakowka S, McCullough B, Koestner A, Olsen R (1973) Myelin specific autoantibodies associated with central nervous system demyelination in canine distemper virus infection. Infect Immun 8:819–827

Kristensson K, Wisniewski HM (1977) Chronic relapsing experimental allergic encephalomyelitis. Studies in vascular permeability changes. Acta Neuropathol 39:189–194

Kristensson K, Wisniewski HM, Bornstein MB (1976) About demyelinating properties of humoral antibodies in experimental allergic encephalomyelitis. Acta Neuropathol 36:307–314

Krücke W (1973) On the histopathology of acute hemorrhagic leucoencephalitis, acute disseminated encephalitis and concentric sclerosis. International symposium on aetiology and pathogenesis of the demyelinating diseases, Kyoto, pp 11–27

Lamoureux G, Borduas AG (1966) Immune studies in multiple sclerosis. Clin Exp Immunol 1:363–376

Lampert PW (1965) Demyelination and remyelination in experimental allergic encephalomyelitis. J Neuropathol Exp Neurol 24:371–385

Lampert PW (1967) Electron microscopic studies on ordinary and hyperacute experimental allergic encephalomyelitis. Acta Neuropathol 9:99–126

Lampert PW (1969) Mechanism of demyelination in experimental allergic neuritis. Electron microscopic studies. Lab Invest 20:127–138

Lampert PW, Carpenter S (1965) Electron microscopic studies on the vascular permeability and the mechanisms of demyelination in experimental allergic encephalomyelitis. J Neuropathol Exp Neurol 24:11–24

Lampert PW, Cressman M (1966) Fine structural changes of myelin sheaths after axonal degeneration. Am J Pathol 49:1139–1153

Lampert PW, Kies MW (1967) Mechanism of demyelination in allergic encephalomyelitis of guinea pigs. An electron microscopic study. Exp Neurol 18:210–223

Lassmann G (1969) Beitrag zur Enzymhistochemie der Läsionen bei der multiplen Sklerose des Menschen. Wien Z Nervenheilk [Suppl] II:53–56

Lassmann H, Wisniewski HM (1978) Chronic relapsing EAE. Time course of neurological symptoms and pathology. Acta Neuropathol 43:35–42

Lassmann H, Wisniewski HM (1979a) Chronic relapsing experimental allergic encephalomyelitis. Clinicopathological comparison with multiple sclerosis. Arch Neurol 36:490–497

Lassmann H, Wisniewski HM (1979b) Chronic relapsing experimental allergic encephalomyelitis. Effect of age at the time of sensitization on clinical course and pathology. Acta Neuropathol 47:111–116

Lassmann H, Wisniewski HM (1979c) Chronic relapsing experimental allergic encephalomyelits: Morphological sequence of myelin degradation. Brain Res 169:357–368

Lassmann H, Ammerer HP, Kulnig W (1978a) Ultrastructural sequence of myelin degradation. I. Wallerian degeneration of the rat optic nerve. Acta Neuropathol 44:91–102

Lassmann H, Ammerer HP, Jurecka W, Kulnig W (1978b) Ultrastructural sequence of myelin degradation. II. Wallerian degeneration of the rat femoral nerve. Acta Neuropathol 44:103–109

Lassmann H, Kitz K, Wisniewski HM (1980a) Chronic relapsing experimental allergic encephalomyelitis in rats and guinea pigs – a comparison. In: Boese A. (ed) Search for the cause of MS and other chronic diseases of the central nervous system. Verlag Chemie, Weinheim, pp 96–104

Lassmann H, Kitz K, Wisniewski HM (1980b) Structural variability of demyelinating lesions in different models of subacute and chronic experimental allergic encephalomyelitis. Acta Neuropathol 51:191–201

Lassmann H, Kitz K, Wisniewski HM (1981a) The development of periventricular lesions in chronic relapsing experimental allergic encephalomyelitis. Neuropathol Appl Neurobiol 7:1–11

Lassmann H, Kitz K, Wisniewski HM (1981b) Histogenesis of demyelinated lesions in the spinal cord of guinea pigs with chronic relapsing experimental allergic encephalomyelitis. J Neurol Sci 50:109–121

Lassmann H, Kitz K, Wisniewski HM (1981c) In vivo effect of sera from animals with chronic relapsing experimental allergic encephalomyelitis on central and peripheral myelin. Acta Neuropathol 55:297–306

Lassmann H, Budka H, Schnaberth G (1981d) Inflammatory demyelinating polyradiculitis in a patient with multiple sclerosis. Arch Neurol 38:99–102

Lassmann H, Schwerer B, Kitz K, Egghart M, Bernheimer H (1981e) Pathogenetic aspects of demyelinating lesions in chronic relapsing experimental allergic encephalomyelitis: Possible interaction of cellular and humoral immune mechanisms. Progr Brain Res (in press)

Lassmann H, Kitz K, Wisniewski HM (1981f) Ultrastructural variability of demyelinating lesions in experimental allergic encephalomyelitis and multiple sclerosis. Acta Neuropathol [Suppl] VII:173–175

Lassmann H, Stemberger H, Kitz K, Wisniewski HM (1983) In vivo demyelinating activity of sera from animals with chronic experimental allergic encephalomyelitis. Antibody nature of the demyelinating factor and the role of complement. J Neurol Sci 59:123–137

Lebar R, Boutry JM, Vincent C, Robinaux R, Voisin GA (1976) Studies on autoimmune encephalomyelitis in the guinea pig. II. An in vitro investigation of the nature, properties and specificity of the serum demylinating factor. J Immunol 116:1439–1446

Lebar R, Vincent C, Fischer LeBoubennec E (1979), Studies on autoimmune encephalomyelitis in the guinea pig. III. A comparative study with two autoantigens of central nervous system myelin. J Neurochem 32/1451–1460

Lee JC (1971) Evolution in the concept of the blood brain barrier. In: Zimmerman HM (ed) Progress Neuropathol, vol I. Grune and Stratton, New York, pp 84–145

Lesniowski S (1931) Inflammation de la substance grise du tronc cérébral (polioencephalitis superior et inferior) après vaccination antirabique. J Neurol Psychiatr 31:427–440

Levine S (1970) Presidential address: allergic encephalomyelits: cellular transformation and vascular blockade. J Neuropathol Exp Neurol 29:6–20

Levine S (1971) Relationship of experimental allergic encephalomyelitis to human disease. In: Rowland LP (ed) Immunological disorders of the nervous system. Research publications of the association for research in nervous and mental disease, vol XLIX. Williams and Wilkins, Baltimore, pp 33–50

Levine S (1974) Hyperacute neutrophilic and localized forms of experimental allergic encephalomyelitis: a review. Acta Neuropathol 28:179–189

Levine S, Wenk EJ (1965) A hyperacute form of allergic encephalomyelitis. Am J Pathol 47:61–88

Levine S, Sowinski R (1973) Experimental allergic encephalomyelitis in inbread and outbred mice. J Immunol 110:139–143

Levine S, Sowinski R (1974) Experimental allergic encephalomyelitis in congenic strains of mice. Immunogenetics 1:352–356

Levine S, Sowinski P (1976) Necrotic myelopathy (myelomalacia) in rats with allergic encephalomyelitis treated with tilorone. Am J Pathol 82:381–389

Levine S, Hirano A, Zimmerman HM (1965) Hyperacute allergic encephalomyelitis. Electron microscopic observations. Am J Pathol 47:209–221

Levine S, Hoenig EM, Wenk EJ (1967) Altered distribution of lesions after repeated passive transfers of allergic encephalomyelitis. Proc Soc Exp Biol Med 126:454–458

Levine S, Sowinski R, Shaw CM, Alvord EC Jr (1975) Do neurological signs occur in experimental allergic encephalomyelitis in the absence of inflammatory lesions of the central nervous system? J Neuropathol Exp Neurol 34:501–507

Leyden E (1880) Beiträge zur akuten und chronischen Myelitis. Z klin Med 1:1–26

Link H, Tibbling G (1977) Principles of albumin and IgG analyses in neurological disorders. III. Evolution of IgG. Synthesis within the central nervous system in multiple sclerosis. Scand J Clin Lab Invest 37:397–401

Lipton HL, Dal Canto MC, Friedman A (1980) Recent developments in the biology of Theiler's murine encephalomyelitis viruses. In: Boese E (ed) Search for the cause of MS and other chronic diseases of the central nervous system. Verlag Chemie, Weinheim, pp 214–221

Lipton MM, Freund J (1953) The transfer of experimental allergic encephalomyelitis in the rat by means of parabiosis. J Immunol 71:380–384

Lisak RP (1980) Multiple Sclerosis: evidence for immunopathogenesis. Neurology 30:99–105

London Y (1971) Ox peripheral nerve myelin membrane: Purification and partial characterisation of two basic proteins. Biochem Biophys Acta 249:188–196

Ludwin SK (1978) Central nervous system demyelination and remyelination in the mouse. An ultrastructural study of cuprizone toxicity. Lab Invest 39:597–612

Ludwin SK (1980) Chronic demyelination inhibits remyelination in the central nervous system. An analysis of contributing factors. Lab Invest 43:382–387

Lumsden CE (1970) The neuropathology of multiple sclerosis. In: Vinken PI, Bruyn GW (eds) Handbook of clinical neurology, vol 9. Elsevier, New York, pp 217–309

Lumsden CE (1971) The immunogenesis of the multiple sclerosis plaque. Brain Res 28:365–390

Madrid RE, Wisniewski HM (1978) Peripheral nervous system pathology in relapsing experimental allergic encephalomyelitis. J Neurocytol 7:265–282

Madrid RE, Wisniewski HM (1979) Oligodendroglial membrane abnormalities in relapsing experimental allergic encephalomyelitis. J Neuropathol Exp Neurol 38:331

Madrid RE, Wisniewski HM, Iqbal K, Pullakart RK, Lassmann H (1981a) Relapsing experimental allergic encephalomylitis induced with isolated myelin and with myelin basic protein plus myelin lipids. J Neurol Sci 50:399–411

Madrid RE, Goncerzewicz A, Clausen JT, Wisniewski HM (1981b) Genetic resistence to EAE induction in strain magnum guinea pigs. Morphology and immunology. J Neuropathol Exp Neurol 40:337

Marburg O (1906) Die sogenannte "akute Multiple Sklerose". Jahrb Psychiatrie 27:211–312

Marburg O (1936) Multiple Sklerose. In: v Bumke O, Foerster O (eds) Handbuch der Neurologie, vol 13/2. Springer, Berlin

McAlpine D, Compston ND, Lumsden CE (1955) Multiple sclerosis. Livingston, Edinburgh

McDermott JR, Iqbal K, Wisniewski HM (1977) The encephalitogenic activity and myelin basic protein content of isolated oligodendroglia. J Neurochem 28:1081–1088

McFarlin DE, Blank SE, Kibler RF (1974) Recurrent experimental allergic encephalomyelitis in the Lewis rat. J Immunol 113:712–715

McKeown SR, Allen IV (1978) The cellular origin of lysosomal enzymes in the plaque in multiple sclerosis: a combined histological and histochemical study. Neuropathol Appl Neurobiol 4:471–482

McKeown SR, Allen IV (1979) The fragility of cerebral lysosomes in multiple sclerosis. Neuropathol. Appl Neurobiol 5:405–415

Mehta PD, Lassmann H, Wisniewski HM (1980) Immunoglobulin studies in chronic relapsing experimental allergic encephalomyelitis (R-EAE). In: Boese A (ed) Search for the Cause of MS and other chronic diseases of the central nervous system. Verlag Chemie, Weinheim, pp 105–112

Mehta PD, Lassmann H, Wisniewski HM (1981) Immunologic studies of chronic relapsing EAE in guinea pigs: similarities to multiple sclerosis. J Immunol 127:334–338

Mitchell DN, Goswami KKA, Taylor P, Salsbury AJ, Porterfield JS, Micheletti R, Lange LS, Jacobs JP, Hockely DJ, Taylor-Robinson DA, Huddleston JR, Sipe J, Braheny S, Jensen FC, Mc Millan R, Lampert P, Oldstone MBA (1979) Failure to isolate a transmissible agent from the bone-marrow of patients with multiple sclerosis. Lancet II:415–416

Morgan IM (1946) Allergic encephalomyelitis in monkeys in response to injection of normal monkey cord. J Bacteriol 51:614–615

Mori S, Leblond CP (1970) Electron microscopic identification of three classes of oligodendrocytes and a preliminary study of their proliferative activity in the corpus callosum of young rats. J Comp Neurol 139:1–30

Müller E (1904) Die Multiple Sklerose des Gehirns und Rückenmarks. Fischer, Jena

Mussini JM, Hauw JJ, Escourolle R (1977) Immunofluorescence studies of intracytoplasmic immunoglobulin binding lymphoid cells (CILC) in the central nervous system: report of 32 cases including 19 of multiple sclerosis. Acta Neuropathol 40:227–233

Nagai Y, Momoi T, Saito M, Mitsuzawa E, Ohtani S (1976) Ganglioside syndrome, a new autoimmune neurological disorder, experimentally induced with brain gangliosides . Neurosci Lett 2:107–111

Nagai Y, Sakakibara K, Uchida T (1980) Immunomodulatory roles of gangliosides in EAE and EAN. In: Boese, A (ed) Search for the cause of multiple sclerosis and other chronic diseases of the central nervous system. Verlag Chemie, Weinheim, pp 127–138

Niedieck B (1975) On a glycolipid hapten of myelin. Progr Allergy 18:353–422

Niedieck B, Lohmann U (1981) Effector-target cell interaction of lymph node cells from galactocerebroside-sensitised rats with oligodendrocytes of brain cell cultures. J Neuroimmunol 1:191–194

Ninfo V, Rizzutto N, Terzian H (1967) Assoziazione anatomo-clinical di nevrite ipertrofica e sclerosi a placche. Acta Neurol 22:228–237

Oehmichen M (1978) Mononuclear phagocytes in the central nervous system. Neurology Series, vol 21. Springer, Berlin, Heidelberg, New York

Oehmichen M, Grüninger H, Saebisch R, Narita Y (1973) Mikroglia und Perizyten als Transformationsformen der Blut-Monozyten mit erhaltener Proliferationsfähigkeit. Experimentelle autoradiographische und enzymhistochemische Untersuchungen am normalen und geschädigten Kaninchen- und Rattengehirn. Acta Neuropathol 23:200–218

Ogata J, Feigin I (1975) Schwann cells and regenerated peripheral myelin in multiple sclerosis: an ultrastructural study. Neurology 25:713–716

Oldstone MBA, Dixon FJ (1968) Immunohistochemical study of allergic encephalomyelitis. Am J Pathol 52:251–257

Oppenheim H (1914) Der Formenreichtum der multiplen Sklerose. Dtsch Z Nervenheilk 52:169–239

Oppenheimer DR (1976) Demyelinating diseases. In: Blackwood W, Corsellis JAN (eds) Greenfield's neuropathology. Arnold, London, pp 470–499

Oppenheimer DR (1978) The cervical cord in multiple sclerosis. Neuropathol Appl Neurobiol 4:151–162

Ortiz-Ortiz L, Weigle WO (1976) Cellular events in the induction of experimental allergic encephalomyelitis in rats. J Exp Med 144:604–616

Palade GE, Simionescu M, Simionescu N (1979) Structural aspects of the permeability of the microvascular endothelium. Acta Physiol Scand [Suppl] 463:11–32

Panitch H. Ciccone C (1981) Induction of recurrent experimental allergic encephalomyelitis with myelin basic protein. Ann Neurol 9:433–438

Paterson PY (1960) Transfer of allergic encephalomyelitis in rats by means of lymph node cells. J Exp Med 111:119–135

Paterson PY (1971) The demyelinating diseases: clinical and experimental correlates. In: Samter M (ed) Immunological diseases. Little, Brown, Boston, pp 1269–1298

Paterson PY (1976) Experimental allergic encephalomyelitis: role of fibrin deposition in immunopathogenesis of inflammation in rats. Fed Proc 35:2428–2434

Paterson PY, Jacobs AF, Coia EM (1965) Complement-fixing antibrain antibodies and allergic encephalomyelitis. II. Further studies concerning their protective role. Ann. NY Acad Sci 124:292–298

Perier O, Gregoire A (1965) Electron microscopic features of multiple sclerosis lesions. Brain 88:937–952

Perlmann H, Perlmann P, Schreiber RD, Müller-Eberhard HJ (1981) Interaction of target cell bound C 3 bi and C 3 d with human lymphocyte receptors. Enhancement of antibody mediated cellular cytotoxicity. J Exp Med 153:1592–1603

Pertschuk LP, Cook AW, Gupta J (1976) Measles antigen in multiple sclerosis: identification in the jejunum by immunofluoresecence. Life Sci 19:1603–1608

Peters A (1968) The morphology of axons of the central nervous system. In: Bourne GH (ed) The structure and function of the nervous system, vol I. Academic, New York, pp 142–186

Peters G (1935) Zur Frage der Beziehungen zwischen der disseminierten, nicht eitrigen Enzephalomyelitis und der multiplen Sklerose. Z gesamt Neurol Psychiatr 153:356–384

Peters G (1958) Multiple Sklerose. In: Lubarsch O, Henke F, Rössle R (eds) Handbuch der speziellen pathologischen Anatomie und Histologie, vol 13/2. Springer, Berlin Göttingen Heidelberg, pp 525–602

Peters G (1970) Klinische Neuropathologie. Thieme, Stuttgart

Pette E, Mannweiler K, Palacios O, Mütze B (1965) Phenomena of cell membrane and their possible significance for the pathogenesis of so-called autoimmune disease of the nervous system. Ann NY Acad Sci 122:417–428

Pette H (1928) Über die Pathogenese der multiplen Sklerose. Dtsch Z Nervenheilk 105:76–132

Polan CG, Baker AB (1942) Encephalomyeloradiculitis. J Nerv Ment Dis 96:508–522

Pollard JD, King RHM, Thomas PK (1975) Recurrent experimental allergic neuritis. An electron microscopy study. J Neurol Sci 24:365–383

Pollock M, Calder C, Allpress S (1977) Peripheral nerve abnormality in multiple sclerosis. Ann Neurol 2:41–48

Prineas JW (1975) Pathology of the early lesions in multiple sclerosis. Hum Pathol 6:531–554

Prineas JW (1979) Multiple sclerosis: presence of lymphatic capillaries and lymphoid tissue in the brain and spinal cord. Science 203:1123–1125

Prineas JW, Raine CS (1976) Electron microscopy and immunoperoxidase studies in early multiple sclerosis lesions. Neurology 26:29–32

Prineas JW, Connell F (1978) The fine structure of chronically active multiple sclerosis plaques. Neurology 28:68–75

Prineas JW, Wright RG (1978) Macrophages, lymphocytes and plasma cells in the perivascular compartment in chronic multiple sclerosis. Lab Invest 38:409–421

Prineas JW, Connell F (1979) Remyelination in multiple sclerosis. Ann Neurol 5:22–31

Prineas JW, Raine CS, Wisniewski HM (1969) An ultrastructural study of experimental demyelination and remyelination. III. Chronic experimental allergic encephalomyelitis in the central nervous system. Lab Invest 21:472–482

Putnam TJ (1935) Studies in multiple sclerosis. IV. Encephalitis and sclerotic plaques produced by venular obstruction. Arch Neurol 33:929–940

Raine CS, Bornstein MB (1970a) Experimental allergic encephalomyelitis: an ultrastructural study of experimental demyelination in vitro. J Neuropathol Exp Neurol 29:177–191

Raine CS, Bornstein MB (1970b) Experimental allergic encephalomyelitis: a light and electron microscopic study of remyelination and sclerosis in vitro. J Neuropathol Exp Neurol 29:552–574

Raine CS, Wisniewski HM, Prineas J (1969) An ultrastructural study of experimental demyelination and remyelination. II. Chronic experimental allergic encephalomyelitis in the peripheral nervous system. Lab Invest 21:316–327

Raine CS, Snyder DH, Valsamis MD, Stone SH (1974) Chronic experimental allergic encephalomyelitis in inbred guinea pigs – an ultrastructural study. Lab Invest 31:369–380

Raine CS, Wisniewski HM, Iqbal K, Grundke-Iqbal I, Norton WT (1977) Studies on the encephalitogenic effects of purified preparations of human and bovine oligodendrocytes. Brain Res 120:269–286

Raine CS, Traugott U, Stone SH (1978a) Chronic relapsing experimental allergic encephalomyelitis: CNS plaque development in unsuppressed and suppressed animals. Acta Neuropathol 43:43–53

Raine CS, Traugott U, Stone SH (1978b) Glial bridges and Schwann cell migration during chronic demyelination in the CNS. J Neurocytol 7:541–553

Raine CS, Diaz M, Pakingan M, Bornstein MB (1978c) Antiserum induced dissociation of myelinogenesis in vitro. An ultrastructural study. Lab Invest 38:397–403

Raine CS, Barnett LB, Brown A, Behar T, McFarlin DE, (1980) Neuropathology of experimental allergic encephalomyelitis in inbred strains of mice. Lab Invest 43:150–157

Raine CS, Traugott U, Scheinberg LC, Waltz JM (1981a) Morphologic evidence for the secondary involvement of oligodendrocytes in active multiple sclerosis lesions. J Neuropathol Exp Neurol 40:318

Raine CS, Scheinberg L, Waltz JM (1981b) Multiple sclerosis: oligodendroglia survival and proliferation in an active established lesion. Lab Invest 45:534:546

Rapoport SI (1976) Blood brain barrier in physiology and medicine. Raven, New York

Ravinka L, Rogova V, Lazarenko L (1978) Chronic experimental allergic encephalomyelitis in rhesus monkeys and its modification by treatment. J Neurol Sci 38:281–293

Reese TS, Karnovsky MJ (1967) Fine structural localisation of a blood brain barrier to exogenous peroxidase. J Cell Biol 34:207–217

Reichardt M (1957) Das Hirnödem. In: Lubarsch O, Henke F, Rössle R (eds) Handbuch der speziellen pathologischen Anatomie und Histologie, vol 13/1. Springer, Berlin Göttingen Heidelberg, pp 1229–1252

Ridley A (1963) Localisation of gamma-globulin in experimental encephalomyelitis by the fluorescent antibody technique. Z Immun Allergieforsch 125:173–190

Rindfleisch E (1863) Histologisches Detail zur grauen Degeneration von Gehirn und Rückenmark. Arch Pathol Anat Physiol Klin Med (Virchow) 26:474–483

Rinne UK, Riekkinen PJ, Arstilla AV (1972) Biochemical and electron microscopic alterations in the white matter outside demyelinated plaques in multiple sclerosis. In: Leibowitz U (ed) Progress in multiple sclerosis. Academic, New York, pp 76–98

Rivers TM, Schwendtker FF (1935) Encephalomyelitis accompanied by myelin destruction experimentally produced in monkeys. J Exp Med 61:689–702

Rivers TM, Sprunt DH, Berry GP (1933) Observations on attempts to produce acute disseminated encephalomyelitis in monkeys. J Exp Med 58:39-53

Roboz-Einstein E, Robertson DM, Di Caprio JM, Moore W (1962) The isolation from bovine spinal cord of a homogenous protein with encephalitogenic activity. J Neurochem 9:353–361

Roizin L (1949) Histopathologic and histometabolic correlations in some demyelinating diseases. J Neuropathol Exp Neurol 8:381–398

Rorke LB, Iwasaki Y, Koprowski H, Wroblewska Z, Gilden DH, Waren KG, Lief FS, Hoffman S, Cummins LB, Rodriguez AR, Kalter SS (1979) Acute demyelinating disease in a chimpanzee three years after inoculation of brain cells from a patient with MS. Ann Neurol 5:89–94

Rossolimo GJ (1904) Multiple Sclerose. In: Flatau E, Jacobsohn L, Minor L (eds) Handbuch der Pathologischen Anatomie des Nervensystems. Karger, Berlin, pp 691–698

Saida T, Abramsky O, Silberberg DH, Pleasure D, Manning M (1977) Antioligodendrocyte serum demyelinates cultured CNS tissue. Soc Neurosci Abst 7:527

Saida T, Saida K, Dorfman S, Brown NJ, Lisak RP, Manning M, Silberberg DH (1978a) Experimental allergic neuritis (EAN) induced by sensitization with galactocerebroside. J Neuropathol Exp Neurology 37:685

Saida K, Saida T, Brown MJ, Silberberg DH, Asbury AK (1978b) Antiserum mediated demyelination in vivo. A sequential study using intraneural injectin of experimental allergic neuritis serum. Lab Invest 39:449–462

Saida K, Saida T, Brown MJ, Silberberg DH (1979a) In vivo demyelination induced by intraneural injection of anti-galactocerebroside serum. A morphologic study. Am J Pathol 95:99–110

Saida T, Saida K, Dorfman SH, Silberberg DH, Sumner AJ, Manning MC, Lisak RP, Brown MJ (1979b) Experimental allergic neuritis induced by sensitization with galactocerebroside. Science 204:1103–1106

Saida T, Saida K, Brown MJ, Silberberg DM (1979c) Peripheral nerve demyelination induced by intraneural injection of experimental allergic encephalomyelitis serum. J Neuropathol Exp Neurol 38:498–518

131

Schilder P (1912) Zur Kenntnis der sogenannten diffusen Sklerose (über Encephalitis periaxialis diffu-
sa). Z Gesamt Neurol Psychiatr 10:1-60

Schob F (1923) Über Wurzelfibromatose bei multipler Sklerose. Z Gesamt Neurol Psychiatr 83:481-496

Schoene WC, Carpenter S, Behan PO, Geschwind N (1977) Onion bulb formation in the central and
peripheral nervous system in association with multiple sclerosis and hypertrophic polyneuropathy.
Brain 100:755-773

Schwerer B, Lassmann H, Kitz K, Bernheimer H, Wisniewski HM (1981a) Fractionation of spinal cord
tissue affects its activity to induce chronic relapsing experimental allergic encephalomyelitis. Acta
Neuropathol [Suppl] 7:165-168

Schwerer B, Lassmann H, Bernheimer H (1981b) Serum antibodies against CNS antigens in chronic relapsing experimental allergic encephalomyelitis. 8th Int Congress Neurochem, Nottingham, p 266
(abstract)

Seil FJ, Agrawal HC (1980), Myelin proteolipid protein does not induce demyelinating or myelination
inhibiting antibodies. Brain Res 194:273-277

Seil FJ, Falk GA, Kies MW, Alvord EC (1968) In vitro demyelinating activity of serum of guinea pigs sensitized with whole CNS tissue and with purified encephalitogen. Exp Neurol 22:545-555

Seil FJ, Rauch HC, Einstein ER, Hamilton AE (1973) Myelination inhibition factor: its absence in sera
from subhuman primates sensitized with myelin basic protein. J Immunol 111:96-100

Seil FJ, Smith ME, Leiman AL, Kelly JM (1975) Myelination inhibiting neuroelectric blocking factors in
experimental allergic encephalomyelitis. Science 187:951-953

Seil FJ, Quarles RH, Johnson D, Brady RO (1981) Immunisation with purified myelin associated glycoprotein does not evoke myelination inhibiting or demyelinating antibodies. Brain Res 209:470-475

Seitelberger F (1960) Histochemistry of demyelinating diseases proper including allergic encephalomyelitis and Pelizaues-Merzbacher's disease. In: Cumings JN (ed) Modern scientific aspects of neurology. Arnold, London, pp 146-185

Seitelberger F (1967) Autoimmunologische Aspekte der Entmarkungsenzephalitiden. Nervenarzt
38:525-535

Seitelberger F (1973) Pathology of multiple sclerosis. Ann Clin Res 5:337-344

Seitelberger F, Jellinger K, Tschabitscher H (1958) Zur Genese der akuten Entmarkungsenzephalitis.
Wien Klin Wochenschr 70:453-459

Server AC, Lefkowith J, Braine H, McKhann GM (1979) Treatment of chronic relapsing inflammatory
polyradiculoneuropathy by plasma exchange. Ann Neurol 6:258-261

Sever JL, Madden DL (1980) Viruses that do not cause multiple sclerosis. In: Boese A (ed) Search for the
cause of multiple sclerosis and other chronic diseases of the central nervous system. Verlag Chemie,
Weinheim, pp 414-424

Shiraki H (1968) The comparative study of rabies postvaccinial encephalomyelitis and demyelinating en-
cephalomyelitides of unknown origin with special reference to Japanese cases. In: Bailey OT, Smith
DE (eds) The central nervous system: some experimental models of neurological diseases.
Williams and Wilkins, Baltimore, pp 87-123

Shiraki H, Otani S (1959) Clinical and pathological features of rabies post vaccinial encephalomyelitis.
In: Kies MW, Alvord EC (eds) Allergic encephalomyelitis. Thomas, Springfield, pp 58-129

Siemerling E, Raecke E (1914) Beitrag zur Klinik und Pathologie der multiplen Sklerose mit besonderer
Berücksichtigung ihrer Pathogenese. Arch Psychiatr Nervenkr 53:385-564

Silberberg DH, Saida T, Abramsky O, Saida K, Lisak RP, Pleasure D (1980) Approaches to understanding the role of antibody in multiple sclerosis: In: Bauer HJ, Poser S, Ritter G (eds) Progress in multiple
sclerosis research. Springer, Berlin Heidelberg New York, pp 216-220

Simionescu N, Simionescu M, Palade GE (1978) Open junctions in the endothelium of the postcapillary
venoles of the diaphragm. J Cell Biol 79:27-44

Simon J, Anzil AP (1974) Immunhistological evidence of perivascular localisation of basic protein in early development of experimental allergic encephalomyelits. Acta Neuropathol 27:33-42

Simon J, Simon O (1975) Effect of passive transfer of anti brain antibodies to a normal recipient. Exp
Neurol 47:523-534

Simpson JF, Tourtellotte WW, Kokmen E, Parker JA, Itabashi HH (1969) Fluorescent proteins tracing
in multiple sclerosis brain tissue. Arch Neurol 20:373-377

Sluga E (1969) Beitrag zur Feinstruktur der Läsionen bei der multiplen Sklerose des Menschen. Wien Z
Nervenheilk [Suppl] II:59-69

Sluga E (1979) Ultrastruktur der multiplen Sklerose. In: Schmidt RM (ed) Multiple Sklerose, Epidemiologie, Immunologie, Ultrastruktur. Fischer, Jena, pp 261-297

Smith ME (1977) The role of proteolytic enzymes in demyelination in experimental allergic encephalomyelitis. Neurochem Res 2:233-246

132

Smith ME (1980) Proteinase inhibitors and the suppression of EAE. In: Davison AN, Cuzner ML (eds) The suppression of experimental allergic encephalomyelitis and multiple sclerosis. Academic, New York, pp 211–226

Smith SB, Waksman BH (1969) Passive transfer and labelling studies on the cell infiltrate in experimental allergic encephalomyelitis. J Pathol 99:237–244

Snyder DH, Valsamis VD, Stone SH, Raine CS (1975a) Progressive demyelination and reparative phenomena in chronic experimental allergic encephalomyelitis. J Neuropathol Exp Neurol 34:209–221

Snyder DH, Hirano A, Raine CS (1975b) Fenestrated CNS blood vessels in chronic experimental allergic encephalomyelitis. Brain Res 100:645–649

Spielmeyer W (1922) Histopathologie des Nervensystems. Springer, Berlin

Steck AJ, Tschannen R, Schaefer R (1981) Induction of anti-myelin and anti-oligodendrocyte antibodies by vaccinia virus: experimental studies in the mouse. J Neuroimmunol 1:117–124

Steiner G (1931) Regionale Verteilung der Entmarkungsherde in ihrer Bedeutung für die Pathogenese der multiplen Sklerose. In: Krankheitserreger und Gewebsbefund bei multipler Sklerose. Springer, Berlin, pp 108–120

Stochdorph O, Meessen H (1957) Die arteriosklerotische und hypertonische Hirnerkrankung. In: Lubarsch O, Henke F, Rössle R (eds) Handbuch der speziellen pathologischen Anatomie und Histologie, vol XIII/1. Springer, Berlin Göttingen Heidelberg, pp 1465–1510

Stone SH, Lerner EM (1965) Chronic disseminated allergic encephalomyelitis in guinea pigs. Ann NY Acad Sci 122:227–241

Stone SH, Lerner EM, Goode JH (1968) Adoptive autoimmune encephalomyelitis in inbred guinea pigs: Immunological and histological aspects. Science 159:995–997

Stone SH, Lerner EM, Goode JH (1969) Acute and chronic autoimmune encephalomyelitis: age, strain and sex dependency. The importance of the source of antigen. Proc Soc, Biol Med 132:341–344

Strähuber A (1903) Über Degenerations- und Proliferationsvorgänge bei multipler Sklerose des Nervensystems, nebst Bemerkungen zur Aetiologie und Pathogenese der Erkrankung. Zieglers Beitrag Path Anat Allg Pathol 33:409–480

Suzuki K, Andrews JM, Waltz JM, Terry RD (1969) Ultrastructural studies of multiple sclerosis. Lab Invest 20:444–454

Tabira T, Webster HF, Wray SH (1976) Multiple sclerosis cerebrospinal fluid produces myelin lesions in tadpole optic nerves. N Engl J Med 295:644–649

Tabira T, Itoyama I, Kuroiwa Y (1982) Continous antigenic stimulation in chronic relapsing EAE. Abstr IX int congr neuropath, Vienna, p 134

Tandon DS, Griffin JW, Drachman DB, Price DL, Coyle PI (1980) Studies on the humoral mechanisms of inflammatory demyelinating neuropathies. Neurology 30:362

Tavolato B (1975) Immunoglobulin G distribution in multiple sclerosis brain. An immunofluorescence study. J Neurol Sci 24:1–11

Ter Meulen V, Koprowski H, Iwasaki Y, Kräckell YM, Müller D (1972) Fusion of cultured multiple-sclerosis brain cells with indicator cells: presence of nucleocapsids and virions and isolation of parainfluenza-type virus. Lancet II:1–5

Thomas PK, Sheldon H (1964) Tubular arrays derived from myelin breakdown during Wallerian degeneration of peripheral nerves. J Cell Biol 22:715–718

Tourtellotte WW (1970) On cerebrospinal fluid immunoglobulin-G (IgG) quotients in multiple sclerosis and other diseases. J Neurol Sci 10:279–304

Tourtellotte WW, Ma BI (1978) Multiple sclerosis: the blood brain barrier and the measurement of de novo central nervous system IgG synthesis. Neurology 28:76–83

Tourtellotte WW, Potvin AR, Potvin JH, Ma BI, Baumhefner RW, Syndulko K (1980) Multiple sclerosis de novo central nervous system IgG synthesis: measurement, antibody profile, significance, eradication and problems. In: Bauer HJ, Poser S, Ritter G (eds) Progress in multiple sclerosis research. Springer, Berlin Heidelberg New York, pp 106–116

Traugott U, Stone SH, Raine CS (1978) Experimental allergic encephalomyelitis: migration of early T cells from the circulation to the CNS. J Neurol Sci 36:55–61

Traugott U, Stone SH, Raine CS (1979) Chronic relapsing experimental allergic encephalomyelitis: correlation of circulating lymphocyte fluctuation with disease activity in suppressed and unsuppressed animals. J Neurol Sci 41:17–29

Traugott U, Raine CS, Stone SH, Chiba J, Shevach E (1981) Experimental allergic encephalomyelitis: demonstration of T-cells within the CNS using monoclonal antibodies. J Neuropathol Exp Neurol 40:320

Traugott U, Shevach E, Chiba J, Stone SH, Raine CS (1982a) Chronic relapsing experimental allergic encephalomyelitis: Identification and dynamics of T and B cells within the central nervous system. Cell Immunol 68:261–275

Traugott U, Raine CS (1982b) Localisation of T and B cells in multiple sclerosis plaques. Abstr IX, Int Congr Neuropath, Vienna, p 103

Turnbull HM, Mc Intosh J (1926–27) Encephalomyelitis following vaccination. Br J Exp Path 7:181–222

Uchimura I, Shiraki H (1957) A contribution to the classification and the pathogenesis of demyelinating encephalomyelitis. J Neuropathol Exp Neurol 16:139–208

Van Deus B (1977) Vesicular transport of horseradish peroxidase from the brain to blood in segments of the cerebral microvasculature in adult mice. Brain Res 124:1–8

Van Deurs B, Amtorp O (1978) Blood brain barrier in rats to the hemepeptide microperoxidase. Neuroscience 3:737–748

Vandvik B, Reske-Nielsen E (1972) Immunochemical and immunohistochemical studies of brain tissue in subacute sclerosing panencephalitis and multiple sclerosis. Acta Neurol Scand [Suppl] 51:413–416

Van Gehuchten P (1966) Lesions de ganglions spineaux dans la sclerose en plaques. Acta Neurol Belg 66:331–340

Vaughn JE, Hinds PL, Skoff RP (1970) Electron microscopic studies of Wallerian degeneration in rat optic nerves. I. The multipotential glia. J Comp Neurol 140:175–206

Vorbrodt AW, Lassmann H, Wisniewski HM Lossinsky AS (1981) Ultracytochemical studies of the blood-meningeal barrier (BMB) in rat spinal cord. Acta Neuropathol 55:113–123

Wagner HJ, Pilgrim C, Brandl J (1974) Penetration and removal of horseraddish peroxidase injected into the cerebrospinal fluid: role of cerebral perivascular spaces, endothelium and microglia. Acta Neuropathol. 27:299–315

Waksman BH (1959) Activity of proteolipid containing fraction of nervous tissue in producing experimental "allergic" encephalomyelitis. In: Kies MW, Alvord EC Jr (eds) Allergic encephalomyelitis. Thomas, Springfield

Waksman BH (1960a) Experimental study of diphtheric polyneuritis in the rabbit and guinea pig. III. The blood nerve barrier in the rabbit. J Neuropathol Exp Neurol 20:35–77

Waksman BH (1960b) The distribution of experimental autoallergic lesions. Its relation to the distribution of small veins. Am J Pathol 37:673–693

Waksman BH (1980) Introduction to session V. In: Boese A (ed) Search for the cause of multiple sclerosis and other chronic diseases of the central nervous system. Verlag Chemie, Weinheim, pp 371–373

Waksman BH, Adams RD (1962) A histologic study of the early lesions in experimental allergic encephalomyelitis in the guinea pig and rabbit. Am J Pathol 41:135–153

Waksman BH, Morrison LR (1951) Tuberkulin type sensitivity to spinal cord antigen in rabbits with isoallergic encephalomyelitis. J Immunol 66:421–444

Watanabe R, Wege H, Ter Meulen V (1982) Corona virus-host relationship in demyelinating encephalomyelitis of rats: analysis of CMI reactions to myelin and viral antigens. Abstr IX Int Congr Neuropath, Vienna, p 99

Westergaard E (1975) Enhanced vesicular transport of exogenous peroxidase across cerebral vessels induced by serotonin. Acta Neuropathol 32:27–42

Westergaard E, Brightman MW (1973) Transport of proteins across normal cerebral arterioles. J Comp Neurol 152:17–24

Williams RM, Krakowka S, Koestner A (1980) In vivo demyelination by anti-myelin antibodies. Acta Neuropathol 50:1–8

Wisniewski HM, Raine CS (1971) An ultrastructural study of experimental demyelination and remyelination. V. Central and peripheral nervous system lesions caused by diphtheria toxin. Lab Invest 25:73–80

Wisniewski HM, Bloom BR (1975) Primary demyelination as a nonspecific consequence of a cell mediated immune reaction. J Exp Med 141:346–359

Wisniewski HM, Keith AB (1977) Chronic relapsing experimental allergic encephalomyelitis – an experimental model of multiple sclerosis. Ann Neurol 1:144–148

Wisniewski HM, Prineas J, Raine CS, (1969) An ultrastructural study of experimental demyelination and remyelination in the peripheral and central nervous system. I. Acute experimental allergic encephalomyelitis. Lab Invest 21:105–118

Wisniewski HM, Raine CS, Kay WJ (1972) Observations on viral demyelinating encephalomyelitis canine distemper. Lab Invest 26:589–599

Wisniewski HM, Madrid RE, Lassmann H, Deshmukh DS, Iqbal K (1980a) Search for antigen(s) and immunological mechanisms responsible for extensive demylination and relapses in experimental allergic encephalomyelitis. In: Boese A (ed) Search for the cause of multiple sclerosis and other chronic diseases of the central nervous system. Verlag Chemie, Weinheim, pp 89–95

Wisniewski HM, Brosnan CF, Bloom BR (1980b) Bystander and antibody dependent cell-mediated demyelination. In: Davison AN, Cuzner MC (eds) The suppression of experimental allergic encephalomyelitis and multiple sclerosis. Academic, London, pp 45–58

Wisniewski HM, Lassmann H, Brosnan CF, Mehta PD, Lidsky AA, Madrid RE (1982) Multiple sclerosis: immunological and experimental aspects. In: Matthews WB, Glaser GH (eds) Recent advances in clinical neurology, vol 3. Churchill-Livingstone, London, pp 95–124

Wolf A, Kabat EA, Bezer AE (1947) The pathology of acute disseminated encephalomyelitis produced experimentally in the rhesus monkey and its resemblance to human demyelinating disease. J Neuropathol Exp Neurol 6:333–356

Wolfgram F (1979) What if multiple sclerosis isn't an immunological or a viral disease? The case for circulating toxin. Neurochem. Res 4:1–14

Wüthrich R (1980) CT-scan in the diagnosis and assessment of the course of MS. In: Bauer HJ, Poser S, Ritter G (eds) Progress in multiple sclerosis research. Springer, Berlin Heidelberg New York, pp 596–598

Yasuda T, Tsumita T, Nagai Y (1975) Enhancement of encephalitogenic activity by the formation of myelin basic protein acidic protein complex. Jpn J Exp Med 45:415–422

Yokoyama M, Trams EG, Brady RO (1962) Sphingolipid antibodies in sera of animals and patients with central nervous system lesions. Proc Soc Exp Biol Med 111:350–352

Yonezawa T, Ishihara Y, Matsuyama H (1968) Studies on experimental allergic peripheral neuritis. I. Demyelinating patterns in vitro. J Neuropathol Exp Neurol 27:453–463

Yonezawa T, Arizono N, Hasegawa M, Yamamura Y, Miyaji H (1980) In vitro demyelination by lymphocytes and lymphokines from patients and experimental animals. In: Bauer HJ, Poser S, Ritter G (eds) Progress in multiple sclerosis research. Springer, Berlin Heidelberg, New York, pp 67–72

Experimental Brain Research

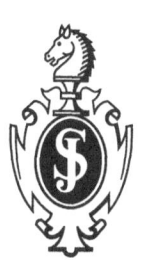

Springer-Verlag
Berlin
Heidelberg
New York
Tokyo

Supplement 1:
Afferent and Intrinsic Organization of Laminated Structures in the Brain
(7th International Neurobiology Meeting)
Editor: O. Creutzfeldt
1976. 127 figures. XXIII, 579 pages
ISBN 3-540-07923-8

Supplement 2:
Hearing Mechanisms and Speech
EBBS-Workshop, Göttingen, April 26–28, 1979
Editors: O. Creutzfeldt, H. Scheich, C. Schreiner
1979. 85 figures, 12 tables. XXIII, 413 pages
ISBN 3-540-09655-8

Supplement 3:
Gonadal Steroids and Brain Function
IUPS-Satellite-Symposium, Berlin, July 10–11,1980
Editors: W. Wuttke, R. Horowski
1981. 136 figures, 10 tables. XIII, 373 pages
ISBN 3-540-10606-5

Supplement 4:
The Renin Angiotensin System in the Brain
A Model for the Synthesis of Peptides in the Brain
Editors: D. Ganten, M. Printz, M. I. Phillips, B. A. Schölkens
1982. 108 figures, 46 tables. XVII, 385 pages
ISBN 3-540-11344-4

Supplement 5:
The Aging Brain
Physiological and Pathophysiological Aspects
Editor: S. Hoyer
1982. 52 figures, 66 tables. XIV, 281 pages
ISBN 3-540-11394-0

Supplement 6:
The Cerebellum – New Vistas
Editors: S. L. Palay, V. Chan-Palay
1982. 264 figures, 16 tables. XVII, 637 pages
ISBN 3-540-11472-6

Supplement 7:
Neural Coding of Motor Performance
Editors: J. Massion, J. Paillard, W. Schultz, M. Wiesendanger
1983. 88 figures, 7 tables. XI, 348 pages
ISBN 3-540-12140-4

E. Braak

On the Structure of the Human Striate Area

1982. 44 figures. VI, 87 pages. (Advances in Anatomy, Embryology and Cell Biology, Volume 77)
ISBN 3-540-11512-9

Adrenal Actions on Brain

Editors: D. Ganten, D. Pfaff
1982. 25 figures. V, 153 pages. (Current Topics in Neuroendocrinology, Volume 2)
ISBN 3-540-11126-3

W. Birkmayer, P. Riederer

Parkinson's Disease

Biochemistry, Clinical Pathology, and Treatment

Translated by G. Reynolds with the assistance of K. Blau and L. Reynolds
With a Foreword by M.D. Yahr
1983. 57 figures. XIII, 194 pages
ISBN 3-211-81722-0

Brain Abscess and Meningitis Subarachnoid Hemorrhage: Timing Problems

Editors: W. Schiefer, M. Klinger, M. Brock
1981. 219 figures, 134 tables. XIX, 519 pages.
(Advances in Neurosurgery, Volume 9)
ISBN 3-540-10539-5
Distribution rights for Japan: Nankodo Co. Ltd., Tokyo

Experimental and Clinical Neuropathology

Proceedings of the First European Neuropathology
Meeting, Vienna, May 6–8, 1980

Editors: K. Jellinger, F. Gullotta, M. Mossakowski
1981. 210 figures. XI, 409 pages. (Acta Neuropathologica, Supplementum 7)
ISBN 3-540-10449-6

R. Nieuwenhuys, J. Voogd, C. van Huijzen

The Human Central Nervous System

A Synopsis and Atlas

2nd revised edition. 1981. 154 figures. VIII, 253 pages
ISBN 3-540-10316-3
Distribution rights for Japan:
Igaku Shoin Ltd., Tokyo
Also available in German

A.M. Neville, M.J. O'Hare

The Human Adrenal Cortex

Pathology and Biology – An Integrated Approach

1982. 173 figures. XIV, 354 pages
ISBN 3-540-11085-2

M. Swash, M.S. Schwartz

Neuromuscular Diseases

A Practical Approach to Diagnosis and Management
1981. 167 figures. XXII, 316 pages
ISBN 3-540-10548-4

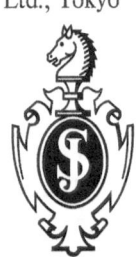
Springer-Verlag Berlin Heidelberg New York Tokyo